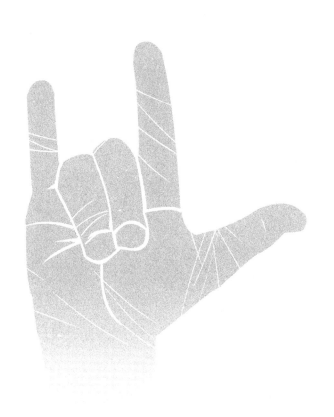

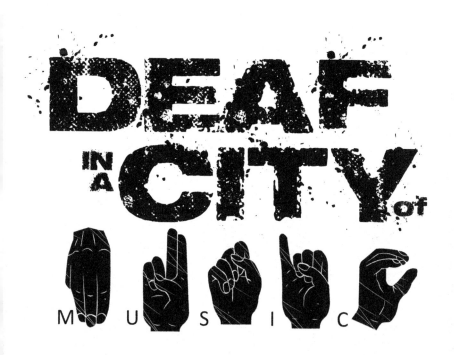

POPPY O'GUIN STEELE

GOLDMINDS

NASHVILLE, TENNESSEE

Deaf in a City of Music
ISBN 13: 978-1-942905-35-6
Library of Congress control number: 2011928604

Cover design by Brenda Bradshaw, Travis Hanson, & Stacy Sheppard

Goldminds Publishing, LLC.
1050 Glenbrook Way, Suite 480
Hendersonville, TN 37075

www.goldmindspub.com

Dedicated to the Creator of small, smooth stones.

Table of Contents

Prologue

My Playlist (a disclaimer)

No perfect person lives here. Not even close. My mouth is a size 8 ½ in women's shoes. I mean well, but words come out of my mouth the wrong way. I forget important dates of family and friends. I write down their birthdates and anniversaries, but life happens and they slip by. I have wardrobe malfunctions. I trip and stumble. I feel awkward at frou-frou events. I am not perfect.

So, I do not pass judgment on others. I do not preach to anyone… except my children. I get by the only way I know how, but I never impose my choices on others.

When people ask me (and they frequently do) how I have managed to get through some situations described in the following pages, I say "only by the grace of God." I have literally survived on a wing and a prayer for years.

This is my survival playlist. These songs have kept me moving forward. Like many others, music feeds my soul.

"I Will Not Be Moved" by Natalie Grant

"Above It All" by Building 429

"Eagles" by Third Day

"Voice of Truth" by Casting Crowns

"All Right" by MercyMe

"Free to Be Me" by Francesca Batestelli

"He Leadeth Me" by Acapella

Every day I drove to work playing the same song over and over and over. For a few months. And then I changed the song and played it over and over and over again. My children didn't seem to mind, and the constant assurance from the lyrics got me through. When doubt crept in, the "Voice of Truth" reminded me that a power much greater than me had the situation under control. When the people I was trying to work with seemed to be in such a helpless, hopeless state and I wanted to run to a happy place to escape, "Above it All" reminded me it wasn't about me. It was about them. Always.

As Alcoholics Anonymous encourages reliance on a Higher Power, I, too, find strength in my Higher Power, God my Creator. I do not force this on the reader. I only explain how I could get up in the morning and put one foot in front of the other. This is my journey. Not a sermon. Please glean as you wish.

"No one is as deaf as the man who will not listen."
Jewish Proverb

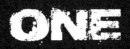

I have Voice. Hear me Roar.

"Hear my words that I might teach you."
Simon and Garfunkel, "The Sounds of Silence"

Music is big business here. Writing it. Singing it. Marketing it. Selling it. Even the practice of medicine in this City of Music is catered to the god, music. Famous musicians have their vocal cords tuned here.

Now, I am not complaining. I love music. I have my iPod and CD holder stocked full of my favorites. I have spent a pretty penny on tickets to see Paul McCartney—three times. But I also work with a population who enjoys music differently than I do. I see what a dichotomy this City of Music is for those who do not hear with their ears but with their eyes. The home of the Great Johnny Cash is not the home to the Great Mindy and Theron.

In this City of Music, deafness is a tragedy in need of a remedy. For this reason, there is a big push for cochlear implants and speech training. And a big discouragement from sign language.

There is nothing wrong with cochlear implants and hearing aids. They are a miracle of technology. They are assistive technology that has made a world of difference for so many. But they are not necessarily the miracle cure that many in the hearing world imagine them to be. Conversations with Deaf adults can shed light on the Deaf perspective. Experience with a cochlear implant simulator can also be quite informative about what the Deaf experience. Accommodations are still needed. Keeping eye contact with those who have cochlear implants and hearing aids is important. Often those with assistive technology enjoy rap music most because of the strong beat and rhythm which is least effected by the difference in sound through technology.

This City of Music is also the Buckle of the Bible Belt. Millions of dollars are spent on international missions and gospel music, Christian books, Christian curriculum. Yet the deaf are the third largest unreached group of people with the gospel. They live next door. And a third-world away.

This is not a gripe session, but an awakening to the abuse and neglect of millions of Americans. Americans who shop in our stores, sit in our classrooms, die in our hospitals, waste away in our prisons.

This is a call to arms to do what is right.

Most people truly want to do what is right. I do honestly believe that. But what is right is frequently uncomfortable and very hard.

It is much easier to go along with the majority and not disturb the status quo. We see evidence of this frequently in the news. Many child abuse cases have been silenced for years because people have been scared to pursue justice. It is easier to cave in. It is hard to stand up for right.

The stories that follow will require some discomfort and inconvenience for some in order to make it right. A chorus of concerned citizens is needed.

Strong to meet the foe, Marching on we go, While our cause we
know Must prevail; /Shield and banner bright Gleaming in the
light, Battling for the right, We ne'er can fail. /Rouse then, Soldiers!
Rally round the banner! Ready, steady, pass the word along; /
Onward, forward, shout aloud…(verse 2).
William F. Sherwin, 1869, "Sound the Battle Cry"

~ ~ ~

One day when I was about nine years old, I had a brush with death. It was my first day at an after school program. My new set of friends and I were playing with a red kickball. As balls always do, it soared over the fence and into the adjoining yard. The group of kids and I lined up along the chain-link fence and peered over the top. I looked down the fence at all of the faces on my right and left and wondered why no one was going to get it. Didn't they know how? Had no one shown them how to clear a fence? Were they waiting for the team captains? If we were waiting for a teacher, then we would waste valuable kickball play time. So I shrugged my shoulders and planted the toes of my tennis shoes one at a time in the small wire-diamond shapes then swung my legs over the top. I hit the green grass solidly with my feet and jogged over to the ball.

Then out of the corner of my eye, I saw a flash of black.

Now in those moments of terror, time slows to comical movie time speed. I don't understand why. Or how.

With that flash of black, I smelled, heard, felt, and saw the presence of a death-eater Doberman that was lightning fast and foaming at the mouth. I was in his yard, and he wanted me to die.

My legs jumped into survival speed. I have never run so fast in all of my life. I reached the ball and threw it over the fence…because getting the ball was the point and it would be a waste if we lost the ball AND I died. Once the ball left my hand, I flew back to the fence and quite possibly cleared it like a hurdle in one big jump. I don't actually remember. But I do remember that as soon as my feet touched the dusty ground back in the safe zone a teacher's hand was on the scruff of my neck and she nearly dragged me to the side of the building where I was made to sit until my mom came to get me. I don't remember if they yelled at me. I know that I didn't cry. Until I got home.

But we got our ball back.

I learned something that day. I learned that I am one of the crazy people who will jump the fence to get the ball. I learned that I can run when I need to. I learned that I will save the ball no matter what. When I was nine, it was a ball. When I was 35, it was a child.

At 35 I saw no one jumping the fence to save the child. Why were they not jumping the fence? Had no one shown them how? So I jumped the fence. Only this time I knew there would be a Doberman. Maybe pit bulls, too. But the child needed to be back in the yard where it belonged. I had to trust that the speed in my legs would return when I needed it. I had to get the child.

Many have called me irrational, illogical, prone to exaggeration, hyper-sensitive, glory-seeking, and child-exploiting. Name calling doesn't change the fact that a child is in someone else's yard in the danger zone. If no one else will go in, I will.

This cloak of responsibility that I feel doesn't seem like it fits me well. My obstacles feel more challenging because "I don't have a dog in this fight". I am neither deaf nor do I have deaf family. That has been a real problem. I have no authority to insist anyone do anything that they should. I am an outsider and yet I am forced to see the world through the eyes of the Deaf. It isn't pretty. I speak these words as a member of the hearing world to the hearing world with all empathy for the Deaf. I have seen how the world can be better. I grew up in it. With a little education, and a little adjustment on the part of the hearing world, this world CAN be a better place for us all. And in this world where we face tornadoes, tsunamis, typhoid and terrorists, wouldn't it be nice to know you have more people on your side fighting the good fight and working to find answers to the greater enemies?

I am not deaf, and I am not a CODA, Child of a Deaf Adult. I am not a parent of a deaf child. I am not even related to a Deaf adult. And this is my story.

Allow me interrupt here to explain "Deaf" and "deaf." Capital "D" "Deaf" refers to the community of people who are identified with the culture of Deaf, who may or may not include people who have cochlear implants, hearing aids, varying degrees of hearing, CODAs and sometimes interpreters. Lower case "d" "deaf" refers to the physical condition relating to hearing. These two spellings serve to communicate huge differences within the Deaf world.

When I was six years old, my mom married the man I call Dad, and we started attending a church with a Deaf congregation. That Deaf congregation had a Deaf preacher and about 30-60 Deaf members. The Deaf congregation met in the fellowship room in metal-framed, plastic chairs on concrete floors. That was significant to a child in Deaf church because the chairs made noise when climbed on, and the floor made noise when pens dropped. My cough during cold season made echo noises. Of course, very few people would have known that, but I was very aware that I was the loudest sound during worship. My parents began interpreting the worship for any hearing people who attended the Deaf service.

A mysterious chain of events led to that.

Dad had a sixteen-year-old son who died in a motorcycle accident when I was eight. My parents had been attending sign language classes and became friends with the Deaf. At my brother's funeral, the Deaf came out in droves because, as is typical of the Deaf Community to those learning their language, they whole-heartedly loved and supported my parents. That show of support really affected my parents, so we never left them. That is when the Deaf World became my world.

My worship services, weddings, potlucks, and funerals were all with the Deaf. They were my church family. Of course, I let my parents interpret for me. It was easier to let someone else do it. I never actually attended sign language classes, but, as children do, I naturally picked up the language. Tuesday nights in my family were silent dinners. My parents only communicated in sign language - regardless of whether we dined in or out. As an adolescent and teenager, I was so embarrassed by that. I was the 'interpreter' for waitresses. Of course, everyone thought they were Deaf and I was a CODA.

I was grateful to go to college and attend worship as normal hearing America. I did not major in interpreting or American Sign Language (ASL) because however much I loved Deaf people and marveled at the beauty of their language, I did not want the isolation that came with the Deaf World. So, I worked in journalism, majored in English and avoided social work classes and psychology classes for self-preservation. I wanted to be Atticus Finch and change the world.

Then I married and moved to Smalltown, America.

In Smalltown, earth-shaking journalism didn't happen. The local paper reported who was late to church on Sunday and whom they sat by. I found a temp job working as a bookkeeper at a construction company. It was like kryptonite. I abhor the mindless tedium and repetitive monotony of numbers. The subcontractors were condescending and arrogant. The construction workers were crass and insulting. I couldn't imagine what purpose I could serve there.

I vividly remember standing in the shower one morning, dreading going to work and weeping. I remember praying, asking God why in the world He had me in this job. I was ready to be Atticus Finch and right all wrongs.

Then one day a subcontractor walked in with his Deaf worker. I signed to the gentleman. He was clearly surprised and asked me how I knew Sign. I told him my story.

He said, "I know that church and the preacher."

"How?" I asked.

"I am a member of the church, too," he replied.

Then it was my turn to be surprised. "Really? Where? I didn't know there was a Deaf church around here!"

"There isn't," he signed. "We don't have an interpreter."

I couldn't believe it. Where I had grown up, we had half-a-dozen interpreters.

I said, "I am not good by any means, but if you want to come to worship, I will do everything I can to help you understand what is going on." He did come. With his Deaf wife. And seven Deaf children. Deaf sisters, brothers-in-law, nieces, grandchildren, friends. Within one year we had twenty-four Deaf members.

A Deaf gentleman and his family showed up at church one Sunday. He said he was a preacher and wondered if the church would be interested in him as the Deaf preacher.

The following Monday morning the pulpit minister called me into his office. He said, "Poppy, where did this man come from? He didn't just fall from the sky!"

I nodded.

"Well, all I can say is someone must have been praying," he said.

I smiled and said, "That would be me."

"Well, I want to talk with him. Can you get him here to have lunch with me? Of course, I will need you to interpret," he said.

A few days later we were at the Dairy Dip for lunch. A three-hour lunch. I interpreted back and forth. My food was never touched because I couldn't eat with my hands full or my mouth full. No complaints. I was just so thrilled to have help coming.

Next we started sign language classes. Forty people from the church showed up. I pushed them hard because I needed help. Eight people stuck with me. None of us were good, but we did our best and the Deaf kept coming.

I started getting calls from various institutions in the county: police, hospitals, funeral homes, courts, child development centers, and schools. They didn't want to pay for a real interpreter and I didn't want the Deaf to go without one. I soon found out what a disservice I was doing to the Deaf community. As long as all of these institutions were getting free services – regardless of the qualifications of the person interpreting – they would never hire a certified interpreter. Deaf history is full of stories about children interpreting for their parents in medical situations where parents suffered because they did not receive clear communication from a qualified professional. How many seven year olds could explain to mom why she needed chemotherapy and the ramifications? Could the seven-year-old even spell chemotherapy? How many children would be able to go with mom to a gynecologist? What mother would want her child there? What the Deaf world needs is access to certified interpreters and solidarity from those of us who love them.

This is where the journey began.

I am a stranger here, within a foreign land; My home is / far away, upon a golden strand; Ambassador to be of / realms beyond the sea, I'm here on business for my King. (verse 1)

E. Taylor Cassel, 1902, "I Am a Stranger Here"

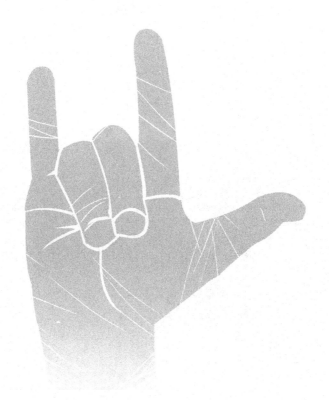

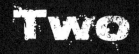

Two

The Police

"We can go on, go on, silent as the tomb/ Let the path of least resistance lead us right back to our rooms…"(lines 4-6).
Michael Higgins, "In This House"

Joey

The first time I went to the police department was for a young man who was scheduled for a plea hearing on his second DUI offense. He had been in jail for a few days and I was his first interpreter. Of course, he hadn't had his first phone call because there was no TTY (This is a now-archaic form of technology that allows a deaf person to type messages through telephone systems to another person or relay site which has TTYs. The person reading the message at the relay site can then speak through the telephone to the hearing person on the other end.) or interpreter, and he didn't know he could demand either or both.

I was so naïve. I had no idea what I was walking into.

Joey walked into the courthouse in orange coveralls and flip-flops. The police removed his handcuffs so that we could talk. Not understanding that he was clueless as to what was going on, I asked him if he would plead guilty or innocent.

He replied, "I am gonna ask the judge if he has a Playboy."
I thought, 'He must not have understood my sign,' and repeated my question.

He shrugged.

'Wow.' I think, 'This is gonna be tough.'

I later learned that Joey was from a school for the Deaf in the North. His signing accent sounded like what I imagined someone from the Bronx sounded like, very low signs, slurred and heavy with attitude.

I sign Southern.

The judge sent him to call his father. Since there is no TTY there, I picked up a phone in the front office and held the receiver to my ear with my shoulder while I signed the conversation with his father. His father said, "Tell the son-of-a-bitch that he should have learned his lesson the first time. I ain't bailing his butt out. He can rot there. I don't care."

Dial tone.

I signed, "He said that you are on your own and he is not coming."

I couldn't bring myself to sign the actual conversation. That was a BIG interpreter error, but then again, I was not a real interpreter. I later learned that during Joey's growing up years, he experienced things like being locked in the back bedroom when company came to visit. Then, like 90% of hearing parents with deaf children, his dad never learned to sign.

When Joey did get out of jail, he came to church. He stayed. He brought his girlfriend to sign language classes. She stayed. A few months later I interpreted their wedding.

The experience at the police department unnerved me. I was in over my head. So I called the Center on Deafness in the Big City and talked with the head of the interpreting department, Suzy.
Suzy emphasized the need for certified interpreters in such instances for the Deaf client, the courts and for my own protection. She emphasized I should not interpret as a "helper" or businesses would never pay for a certified interpreter. I tucked away that information in my mental "file cabinet".

Not long afterward I received a phone call from the police at 2 a.m. A hearing child had been raped, but the child's parents were Deaf.

I was stuck.

What do I do? I knew that rape was time-sensitive. An interpreter from Big City could take hours to arrive, but the law required a certified interpreter, so I told them to call one. They called me back and said that they didn't need me anyway because the child could interpret herself. (Not the right answer, either.)

The next day I called Suzy. She advised me if it happened again to tell the police that they should call an interpreter from Big City, but I could interpret at the hospital until the actual interpreter arrived. If the police asked questions or depositions began, I was to stop interpreting and advise them to wait until the certified interpreter arrived.
The years have seasoned me, and I now have no problem saying those words. Back then I just felt like the enemy for not helping. It is still tough, but I have seen the results of "helping" and realize it isn't helping at all. In 2015, we still have problems getting equal access for our deaf friends.

Rosa Parks sat on a front seat. I can sit on my hands.

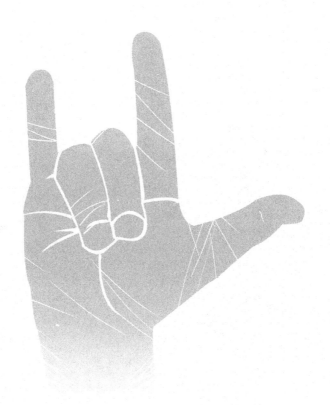

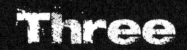

The Funerals

"Now if your spirit's thirsty and your cup is dry/ I know a river where the water is ever sweet/ You've found a friend gonna help you round that bend/You can ride with me."
(lines 11-14)

Michael, Benjamin, and Emily Higgins, "You Can Ride With Me"

One of the early lessons in the School of Hard Knocks came from the funerals I was called to interpret. I cut my teeth on business negotiating, Americans with Disabilities Act (A.D.A.) advocating, deaf family dynamics, and religious doctrine. All of these lessons-learned came at a time when I would have preferred to simply bake a cake for the family, offer hugs and sympathy, and then sit with the friends and family during the memorial service. I felt unqualified for anything else.

Then I remembered the "shower" prayer.

The funerals were very frustrating. The first few called and never paid me. So I billed the next one. $20. I did not ask for money because of the money. Twenty dollars was nothing in the big picture, but it was what I had been advised to do, and I knew it was the right thing to do for the Deaf community. The funeral director refused to pay, saying he couldn't afford it. I knew better. I knew that he pocketed a million a year, and in Smalltown, that is saying something. He had also just constructed a ramp for wheelchairs, but he refused to pay accommodations for the Deaf. He told me that next time he would bill the Deaf family directly. I said, "The A.D.A. specifies accommodations are the responsibility of the public entity."

He said, "I do not have to adhere to the A.D.A. because I have fewer than 15 employees."

Twenty dollars was hardly a hardship for this man, but I am neither a debater nor a negotiator. I let it go. After all, it wasn't my fight. I did not have the power to pursue it. The Deaf have to be the ones to fight. Unfortunately, the word fight sounds very negative and belligerent but after experiencing the constant obstacles, frustrations, and feelings of powerlessness, I start to understand the anger of the Deaf.

But I learned that the Deaf in the area had grown up under such conditions and either didn't know they could fight—and win, didn't know how to fight, or just accepted life as a second-class citizen. Their parents, after all, didn't sign, so they were lacking in many areas of common knowledge.

The only funeral for which I was paid stands out in my memory for different reasons. The lady who had passed away was hearing. Her preacher was hearing. But her children, grandchildren, great-grandchildren and all of their friends and family were Deaf. Nearly all of the full-capacity crowd were Deaf.

Most of the time, in such instances, I prepare what I can ahead of time: music, scriptures, and family names. But this time I had not been able to do so. In fact, I hadn't even met the preacher or known his name.

It was show time. I was in the hallway ready to walk in when the director stopped me and said, "The preacher is refusing to preach the funeral because you are a woman. Apparently, he thinks he is sinning if he shares a pulpit with you."

I had been in Smalltown, in the buckle of the Bible belt, long enough to know that this was a prevalent philosophy. I did not have time to debate it. I kicked into problem-solving mode and thought of 2 possibilities:

1. He could go ahead and preach without an interpreter, but hardly anyone would know what was said—including the entire family.

2. Three Deaf preachers were in attendance, any of whom could preach a funeral at a moment's notice; of course, they hadn't known the deceased.

I was discussing this with the director when one of his colleagues approached us, saying he had convinced the preacher to proceed.

It was a very awkward service. I never actually met the man or had the opportunity to explain the role of an interpreter. Usually, a little explanation of how an interpreter works is sufficient to help people who have problems with what they call a "woman preacher". Normally, I would explain that the gender of a microphone or telephone receiver is as applicable as the gender of the interpreter. The message does not originate with the interpreter. It is a non-issue in the Deaf world. This five-minute discussion normally suffices for smoother relations, but not always. For those others, I have always offered to teach them sign language so that they can interpret themselves. After all, I didn't actually want to be an interpreter myself. In those instances, never has the man accepted my proposal.

There are those with a need. If no one else can or will then, yes, I will. I am satisfied with God as my judge.

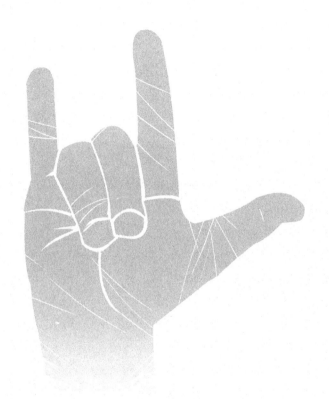

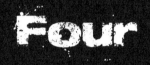

Woman Preacher Problems

"So much of what this life can be/All depends on what you
see." (lines 19-20)
Michael Higgins, "What It Really Is"

Our congregation was planning a big revival in which they invited a big name speaker and launched an advertising campaign. For this special Sunday, the leadership requested that the Deaf combine services with the hearing congregation. The Deaf had many guests coming as well, guests who were traveling from far away.

The guest preacher learned a week before the assembly that I was the interpreter. He refused to preach. The leadership came to me with the problem. My advice was one of two options:

1. They could call Big Town and request a male interpreter.
   (I didn't hold out hope. I knew of none.)

2. Allow the Deaf to have their own service as normal.

The leadership came up with option 3, to which I warned against. Of the eight people who had stuck with me through sign classes, one was a man. His sign skill was about a kindergarten level. I was very proud of his progress, but he was not ready for a platform interpreting assignment in front of highly educated Deaf professionals. Option 3 prevailed. The reaction of the Deaf was predictable and highly toxic. They were insulted and outraged. They had been demoted to second-class Christians. That began the chain of events, which led to disaster. I often felt much like Cassandra in the fall of Troy, who was gifted with the power to foresee the future but cursed in that no one who heard her would believe. I could see what was going to happen, but I was powerless to make it stop.

The leadership commented on how smoothly all had worked out. I countered that the Deaf had been deeply hurt. The leadership response was 'tut-tut. It will be okay.'

It wasn't. Within two years, the Deaf were gone.

On another day the Deaf preacher spoke to the entire congregation, hearing and Deaf. Since I normally voiced for him in Deaf worship, I assumed I would be voicing for him in "big church." I was wrong. While it was a concession to let a woman sign in worship or speak around the Deaf, a woman's voice could not come through the audio system of the main auditorium. Some might be offended. Instead, since the Deaf preacher had the ability to speak, they asked if he would use his voice to speak from the pulpit.

I knew that the leadership was not familiar with the Deaf world and its social norms. I tried my very best to diplomatically educate them without seeming to have authority over them and to tell them what to do. I don't know that I succeeded.

In this case, I explained to the leadership that in the Deaf world to ask a Deaf man to speak was the equivalent of asking a black man to paint his face white, or a white man walking into a black church in black face paint. Asking him to speak was insulting. If he CHOSE to do it, he had that prerogative. We should not ask that. They understood the comparison and heeded my advice.

This time the solution was that I called my dad to come and voice for the preacher. Now, my dad had been signing for about twenty years by this time. He was skilled–with the Deaf with whom he worked. Since I had been voicing for the preacher at our congregation for a while, I had learned all of his nuances and how he preferred to phrase concepts. As skilled as my dad was, he was not the most qualified in this instance. The one to suffer most was the preacher. And then the hearing audience who did not get the full effect of that day's sermon.

I thought back to my childhood. I distinctly remember when a visiting Deaf preacher spoke to the entire 1000-member congregation. His daughter was his official interpreter. Before he spoke, a member of the leadership stood and explained to the congregation what the role of an interpreter was and why they would be hearing the voice of a woman over the sound system. I do not recall ever hearing anyone say they were offended or complain.

I wondered about the thinking processes of the local congregation. My woman's hands were just as female as my woman's voice. Why was one acceptable and the other sinful? And why was my woman's voice acceptable in the Deaf service but not in the hearing service? If one was wrong were not all wrong? One gentleman told me that a woman interpreter did not offend the Deaf because that was all they knew: that they didn't have a choice. He is also one of the men who turned me down for signing lessons. I have never wasted a second on guilt over the decision to interpret in church when no other interpreter was available. The Deaf pity such thinking by hearing individuals. They even have a special sign for the stupidity and superiority of some of the hearing. It is accompanied by eye-rolling.

And here I must address an area that continues to pop up in this journey of finding support and assistance for Deaf children who are abused. I was once approached by a Christian television station about doing an interview about what we do—advocating for deaf children who are abused. The gentleman I spoke with said that he did not believe that abuse was so rampant with the deaf. Who, after all, would hurt a disabled child? He told me to turn in research and a list of experts who would be willing to be interviewed on camera.

So, I set about gathering what he had asked for. I found no Deaf people willing to go on camera to tell their stories (not surprisingly). I did find a PhD in psychology willing to discuss the huge needs for counseling in the Deaf world and the great need for more research among those who are abused. Another expert I had talked with responded by saying that in his many years of working with deaf children who were abused, he found the "church" to be one of the greatest enemies. The "church" frequently covered up abuse, ignored it, or offered prayer as the only weapon to fight it. He asked the motives of the television station, whether they were truly wanting to help or being self-serving…I couldn't honestly answer. He politely declined the invitation. I did find some more willing interviewees and research that I sent. The interview didn't happen.

Through the years I have been called frequently by churches who need interpreters for their worship services. Most of the time they are willing to compensate the interpreter, at least a little. But the largest churches, (the ones where the children pay $800 to go to church camp), have not only refused to pay for interpreters, they have refused use of facilities and equipment. I do not mention these examples of churches involvement as a criticism, but more as a mirror, a request for reflection on what service to the community and heart of missions really means. Pictures of sick children and fly-infested huts in the jungles of Africa are pictures of real needs in this world. Please, send help. By the same thought, a neglected deaf child in Albuquerque is just as worthy of love and attention as one in Africa. We cannot take a picture of the deaf child in Albuquerque, but she is just as real. And if taken care of, the girl from Albuquerque might be the very person to come up with a solution for the children in Africa.

From Greenland's icy mountains, From India's coral strand, Where Afric's sunny/ fountains Roll down their golden sand: From /many'an ancient river, From many'a palmy plain, They call us to deliver Their land from error's chain. (verse 1)
Reginald Heber, 1819, "From Greenland's Icy Mountains"

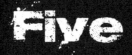

Child Development

"Do my words reach your inner ear/
Or pass through these rafters like I was never here?"
(lines 1-2)
Michael Higgins, "In This House"

Anyone who has ever seen the movie *The Miracle Worker* can appreciate the dedication of those who work with special-needs children every day. Children (and adults) who struggle to communicate their needs and feelings often become behavior problems, and sometimes in their frustration become violent. It is not because they are truly problem individuals, but simply that they long to be understood.

Imagine a child who absolutely abhors peanut butter, yet every day someone continues giving the child a peanut butter sandwich. A child who can communicate that preference will say, "No like!" or "Me no want!" or "I would prefer Grey Poupon with prosciutto, please." If a child struggles with communicating, he or she will begin throwing the peanut butter sandwich, or begin kicking and screaming. The hearing world often interprets this as a behavior problem.

The Child Development Centers (CDC) in Smalltown asked me to come to their facility once a year to teach some basic signs to the teachers who, in turn, would teach the children. They had heard about me, like most places had, because we had a Deaf congregation at our church. We often held free sign language classes at the church for the community. The community quickly learned that when they had a need surrounding the deaf population, they contacted the church. Those needs were as varied as the places and people who called. We were serving adults, children, and various community establishments. The truth is, an oasis in the desert must carry water and food and gasoline and first aid supplies and car repair supplies and baby supplies and bathrooms because it is the only resource to fulfill the needs of those traveling in the wilderness. Such is the life of those who work with the deaf in rural America. We become 'all things to all people' with the common denominator of a need to communicate. Communication is a lifeline. And in this case, the CDC needed communication.

The children at the CDC rarely were deaf or even had any amount of hearing loss. Often the children just had a language delay, which could be caused by a myriad of reasons. So as the teachers began communicating in sign language with the children, the children's frustrations were reduced, and negative behaviors disappeared. Whatever the cause, successful communication improved relationships and learning. That child no longer threw the peanut butter sandwich. Instead, he ate tuna—his favorite. He asked in sign language.

On the first day that I went to the CDC, I realized I had a lot to learn. I had just left a job working in a college classroom which was a stark contrast to children with special needs. The children were autistic. I had never had experience with autistics and suddenly I was in a room with six of them. On the playground, one of the children had green snot that rolled from his nose in a slow ooze. One of the assistants from a nearby classroom suggested to another that they needed to bring out tissues for him. The classroom assistant said, "He'll just eat the tissue. His tongue is catching it anyway."

One day, as I helped with the deaf children, the autistic children in the room started one by one blowing up in screaming tantrums. Within 20 minutes, there was a chorus of screaming, and throwing shoes and projectiles from every corner of the room. They had run out of corners. I remember looking at the face of the deaf child thinking that he was the most content soul in the room. He sat quietly playing as chaos reigned around him.

Once I worked with a child who had cochlear implants yet her parents wanted her to learn sign language for those times when she didn't have the cochlear implant on or when the technology was broken. She would often give herself a time-out in the afternoons because the noise and activity of a room of children was more than she could handle. So she would move to a couch on the opposite side of the room.

One day when she was in her "quiet place" another deaf child walked into the room and asked me a question in sign language. We communicated in sign language for a few moments and the child left. Later that night, the child with cochlear implants told her mom about me and the other deaf child. She asked her mom if that was how the child and I communicated—with our hands? Her mom was shocked that she hadn't connected that before but said yes, that was what sign language was for. The child said, "Wow. That is peaceful."

Out of the mouths of babes.

It is a concept foreign to those of us in the hearing world. We assume that all deaf want to hear and that those who are able to hear after being deaf are overjoyed with their new gift of sound. But the truth is that not all deaf want to hear and not all sound is a blessing. Many deaf prefer to be deaf. Silence can be golden. Sound can be noise. Music through a hearing aid or cochlear implant doesn't sound like the same music through hearing ears. It doesn't mean it is bad. It just means it is different.

I once saw an interview on television where a hearing aid company was giving away hearing aids to a group of deaf/hard of hearing children who couldn't afford them. The reporter asked a child if it was great to hear for the first time. The child was about seven or eight years old and her facial expression was saying that she didn't like what was happening at all. Her nose was crinkling up and her eyebrows were furrowed. She said to the reporter, "Um, not really."

The reporter said, "Of course, it's great!" and laughed as she moved on to more of her report.

The reality is that we in the hearing world do not know what it is like to be in complete silence. No hum from the air conditioner. No birds chirping. No tick of the clock. No swoosh from a passing plane. Total silence. It's peaceful. We in the hearing world do not know what that is. We imagine it to be awful. But that is not necessarily so. It doesn't mean sound is bad. It just means silence is different. Different doesn't have to be bad.

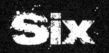

Voc Rehab Work Center

"To love someone more dearly ev'ry day, To help a wand'ring
child to find his way…"(verse 1)
Maude L. Ray, 1903, "My Task

The work center for Vocational Rehabilitation (VR) called me in on an emergency. Like the CDC, they contacted the church. The VR work center hired people with various disabilities to do jobs like pack boxes for companies. They had a Deaf special needs woman, Lorraine, about 20 years old, who was becoming agitated and aggressive because she wasn't being understood. No one on staff and no one in her home knew sign language. They asked me to interpret what she was saying and then teach sign to the staff.

Lorraine was a precious young lady who had Downs Syndrome. She was highly functioning and came from a family who were loving and supportive. They just didn't know sign language. Lorraine was quick with a smile and a hug. She took pride in her tasks and worked very hard.

In the director's office I sat across from Lorraine while the director and teacher observed from the peripheral. Lorraine signed, sloppily but legibly, "February 25, birthday. Want ice cream." It was big. It was loud.

I smiled and said, "FEBRUARY 25 IS MY BIRTHDAY and I WANT ICE CREAM!!"

They laughed, looked relieved, and agreed to get her ice cream.

Belle

"And soon, soon, the melody will come/And note by note the distance is undone/Till the next thing you know, you think you hear someone/Pounding on your walls." (lines 17-20)
Michael Higgins, "In This House"

One Fourth of July I received a call that one of our deaf students who was being serviced by a Vocational Rehabilitation facility did not have family pick her up for the holiday and she had no place to go. My husband and children knew her and agreed that she could spend the holiday with us.

The week proceeded as a normal holiday would until the Fourth.

Traditionally we spend the Fourth at the lake with family, but it was delayed until evening. We were just relaxing by the pool. Then she got on Facebook and saw where her family had posted pictures of celebrating the Fourth without her. She was livid.

Belle stormed into the room where I was and demanded that I

take her to her family. I said, "What are you going to do when you get there?"

She said, "You are going to interpret while I yell at them. Then I am going to throw things at them."

She was weeping and shaking. I had seen her distraught before, but I had never seen anything like this kind of rage.

I said, "I understand you are hurt and angry. That is understandable. But you cannot go over there and throw things at them. What would happen then? Would they call the police?"

"IT IS NOT FAIR!!! IT IS NOT FAIR!!! You will go interpret for me while I yell at them!"

"No." I said. "I cannot do that."

She came up out of her seat towards me. I was frozen where I stood. I couldn't respond to move out of her way.

Thankfully, my husband could. He was immediately in between us. He signed to her, "You cannot do this. We understand you are hurt and angry, but you will not behave this way toward us."

Then my older child got up from the couch and walked the perimeter of the room to avoid where Belle was to get to the bedroom. The look on my son's face cut me to my very soul. He was terrified. No child should have to live like that—scared in his own home. I felt ashamed. I was trying to help abused kids. Kids who lived in fear and my own were now living in fear. I knew then that this could never happen again.

The rest of the holiday was spent counting seconds until it was over. No more angry outbursts, but we refused to bring up the topic of family and kept her as busy as possible.

Patrick

"She knows she will never have money, so she just gives herself/
    And the comfort flows like milk and honey." (lines 7-8)
Michael Higgins and Jeb Stuart Anderson, "Love Ain't Everything"

Some of the sweetest people I have ever known were Deaf. Precious people. One Deaf friend, Patrick, was a roofer who looked like a well-groomed Si Robertson. He was one of seven children, the only deaf. His mother had the German measles while she was pregnant with him, which caused the deafness. He was a graduate of the School for the Deaf and had wanted to go into the army. They don't allow the deaf to enlist.

His skillset included handyman jobs as well as mechanic jobs. One of the stories he loved to tell was once when his car broke down he had gone to a mechanic to get an estimate on fixing it. The mechanic quoted him a price of around $500, which he didn't have. He proceeded to walk to the junkyard, found the part that he needed on an old car, purchased the part for $5 and fixed the car himself.

We hired him to roof our house. He was meticulous. Very good and honest. I remember glancing out a window and seeing him in the yard looking up at the house signing. I looked more closely and realized he was not talking to another Deaf person but to himself. He was counting measurements "out loud" just like anyone else would do.

One day a car pulled up outside while he was roofing and honked its horn. Again. And again. And again. The honk became more irritated with each screech. Finally, a neighbor walked into the street to see what was going on. The red-faced older woman who was behind the wheel bawled out the neighbor because, she said, the rude roofer wouldn't respond when she honked the horn.

The neighbor explained, "He is Deaf, ma'am, and couldn't hear your horn like we could. Can I help you with something?"

She asked for directions then, ashamed, tucked her tail between her legs and sped away.

Patrick never knew.

The most memorable story about Patrick and the roofing involved a ladder. Late one Saturday morning my husband and I had slept in. We had no urgent appointments, so we leisurely arose to prepare breakfast. All the while, we kept hearing something like bees. An odd sound, really. It was intermittent. Distant. Muffled. My husband was curious, so he went to investigate while I cooked. Soon My husband was yelling and running outside, "Patrick is hanging from the second story window ledge!"

The "bees" we heard were Patrick's cries for help while digging his fingers into the window sill. His ladder was flat on the ground. My husband got him down safely.

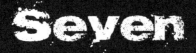

Patrick and I Go Visiting Sandra

"Sometimes the night is like a semicolon/You just got to go
on writing without knowing/Try to find the rhyme and keep
it going/And your options open
Hoping." (lines 11-15)

Michael Higgins, "Semicolon"

Helen Keller once said that blindness separated her from things, but deafness separated her from people. Isolation can be a defining characteristic of the Deaf World. That is why Deaf schools are so revered among the Deaf, why Gallaudet is like Mecca, and why Deaf clubs are a part of every major city. Language is a lifeline. Anyone who has ever traveled in a foreign country and has not been able to speak the language can attest to the relief of hearing someone who does speak the same language as they do.

We tried to reach out to the Deaf in the county, to unite them for the individual's benefit as well as the whole. Together they could be a powerful force.

Patrick and I went to visit a Deaf lady, Sandra, who lived out in the country alone with her five dachshund. It is common for Deaf to have dogs as an alarm system and safety. From the moment I stepped out of the car until the moment we drove off, those five dogs yelped at my feet. Patrick and Sandra were in deep conversation. The incessant barking of the vile creatures didn't bother them. THIRTY SOLID MINUTES. My ears were numb.

Sandra taught me more about the Deaf. One, she told me she was forty years old when she learned how to write a check. Like most Deaf, Sandra's family didn't sign. She had a brother-in-law who felt badly that she always sat alone at family gatherings, so he learned a few signs to use on holidays. One Christmas she took a checkbook to him and asked him to show her how to write it.

Another lesson Sandra taught me about the Deaf experience was more revealing. I had interpreted a funeral for one of her family members. She told me about how the death of her uncle had deeply hurt her and how she had found peace from a box of Cracker Jack's. While she was grieving, she had opened a box and found a plastic white dove as the toy inside. She said that was a sign to her that her uncle was at peace.

I have found that an intriguing belief system is not uncommon in the Deaf world. The Deaf sometimes have very little exposure to communication at all as they are growing up, and when they do it is most often direct orders. For example, one deaf teenager I have worked with was with me in the car when she suddenly turned to me and asked, "What happens to us after we die?" At that moment I was driving in absolute darkness on a winding road. I told her that if I answered right then we might find out very soon the answer to that question.

The gravity of the question in reality hits me to my core because I know that some deaf have no one with whom they can ask those questions. If the family does sign, they sometimes sign things like "go to bed," "get up and get ready," or "clean your plate." The deeper questions of life are never clear for any of us, but for the deaf who can't communicate with anyone around them...they frequently create their own version of what happens based on clues they see around them. Thus, a dove represented Sandra's father at peace.

One day around Christmas time I had a Deaf young lady with me going into church. She looked up at the wall and signed, "OOO! Gross! Who is that guy with blood coming out of his hand?!" I knew that the child had no background in anything religious, but living in the Bible Belt at Christmas time...what did she think of the Nativity scenes? What did she think was the meaning and purpose of that? Without the knowledge of that eternal story, what an absurd tradition that would seem. She lived among Christians and had never heard of Christ.

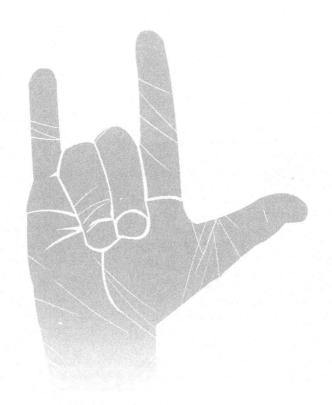

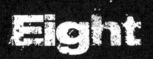

Eight

Neglect

"I was a cool survivor, ran to live, lived to run/Every bruise a badge of honor, every wound a battle won/I didn't know why I was fighting, I only know that now I'm done/All I hear in this silence is 'Follow me, my son'." (lines 1-4)

Michael Higgins and Benjamin Higgins, "This Is The Life"

Bobby's family locked him in the backroom when family came. They were embarrassed by him. Deaf children must be taught that their actions create sounds that can be disturbing to the hearing. That requires patience and communication on the parent's part. For some families, locking the children away is an easier solution.

Bobby was a charmer. He had a boyish face, dimples, and an easy smile. I had a feeling he had met his share of female friends through the years, but I never asked. Bobby met Alicia at a bar. She was hearing and intrigued by Bobby. The two started up a conversation as a sign language lesson.

When Bobby and Alicia were married, Alicia took on the responsibility of filing the taxes. She asked Bobby about his W-2s. He didn't know what she meant. She explained, "You know, what your employers give you at the end of the year so you can file your taxes."

He said, "What do you mean 'file your taxes'?

She said, "You've filed taxes before, right?"

"I don't know what you are talking about!" he said.

Eight years. He had been working for eight years and had never filed his taxes. His family had never talked to him about it. His family had never actually communicated to him in a language he understood—ever.

If the only person in the lives of these Deaf children who can communicate with them in their own language is the interpreter at school, how are the children to learn common knowledge? The interpreter's role is to relate faithfully what is said in the classroom: Science, Social Studies, Math. Deaf education teachers, as all other teachers, are graded on how well their students do on standardized testing. So common knowledge would not be an item that they would be charged with teaching. If parents don't, then who does?

In Bobby's case, his wife did.

Over 95 % of deaf children have hearing parents.
(Mitchell and Karchmer. 2004).
Only 27% of deaf have families who sign at home.
(Gallaudet Research Institute, 2003).

In the Deaf world, like with many minorities, marrying outside of the minority is often frowned upon. So Alicia learned at a Deaf party that she was not welcomed by all Deaf. She said that a Deaf man came up to her and asked if she was hearing. She smiled and nodded yes. He put the palm of his hand in her face and walked away. He did not accept her. That is something that the hearing world has difficulty comprehending, but when one can look at Deaf culture as a minority culture, it begins to match social rules we have already seen established.

Anne

"When the sun comes up on the Fourth Street Mission
There's an angel in an apron in the kitchen
With hands to work and a heart to listen, with a smile." (lines1-3)
Michael Higgins and Jeb Stuart Anderson, "Love Ain't Everything"

My interpreter friends and I have often said that all Deaf children should be born into loving, nurturing homes. For the Deaf children who are not, the struggle to communicate in addition to dysfunction seems like a grossly unfair disadvantage.

Anne is one such case. She is a Deaf lady—a sweet, gentle soul. She speaks so lovingly of her mother who tended so faithfully to her flowerbeds. After her passing, Anne took over. I have never been in her home when the yard and hedges weren't perfectly manicured or the throw pillows fluffed and perched on the sofa or every sugar granule swiped from the kitchen table the second it fell from the spoon. I think she took pride in those tasks, felt peace and comfort, because they connected her to her mother. Every time I saw her, her clothes were neat and her hair tidy. Her eyes were framed by thick black mascara, always reminding me of the Raggedy Ann dolls.

Though neat, her home and clothes always smelled of mildew because the house had drainage issues. Plumbing and construction were not in Anne's skill-set. She lived with her alcoholic father and teenaged daughter, both hearing. I had long suspected that Anne was bullied and/or abused by one or both. She didn't drive or work outside the home. Her daughter was in and out of juvenile correctional facilities. When we had potlucks at church, Anne would ask her ride to wait till the end so she could take the leftovers home with her.

I was worried about her on multiple levels. I talked to her about plans, her future, a job, learning to drive. She always made excuses or delayed. I even sat up an appointment with the vocational rehabilitation center to evaluate her skills and help her get training. She wouldn't go.

Since then, I have learned a lot about victims of domestic violence. It takes an average of seven times for a woman to leave an abusive relationship.

Buck

"Love ain't everything, but it's a place to start/
Such a precious thing to an empty heart." (lines 10-11)
Michael Higgins and Jeb Stuart Anderson,
"Love Ain't Everything"

In rural counties it is not uncommon for the Deaf to have no contact with anyone for long periods of time, much less contact with other Deaf. They will stay in those situations because it is all they have ever known, especially if they did not attend a school for the Deaf. Buck was one of these Deaf. He was a farmer. He grew up on the family farm and learned the trade from his father, as his father had before him. He did know sign language, but he was rarely around anyone who signed. He heard about our deaf congregation through the grapevine...which took a while to reach him...but he sought us out and met us at one of our Silent Dinners.

Silent Dinners are common in larger cities. The Deaf will choose a mall food court or designate a Deaf-friendly restaurant to all meet at once a month. Larger cities will also have Deaf Club bowling nights or movie nights. It helps movie theaters to have all of the deaf come together; then they can turn on the closed-captioning for the whole audience. For Smalltown, we just had a potluck dinner once a month.

Those potlucks were special because it gave the Deaf a private environment where they felt free to be themselves. They would tell jokes and even perform ABC Stories or Deaf dramas. An ABC story or a number story is a story told using the hand shapes for the alphabet or the numbers. One of my favorite ABC stories is an old cowboy who rides into town and stops at a saloon where

35

he has a shoot out. The story begins with the A shape and ends with the Z shape. One popular ABC story is the "Getting Ready in the Morning" story. One Deaf couple created a story like that where he got ready like a man and she got ready like a woman. His G and H might be a razor shaving his face while hers were shaving her legs. You get the idea. In their own environment, the Deaf feel uninhibited and can really tell some funny, funny stories.

So it was at these events that Buck would come out of the woodwork to enjoy food and fellowship. I don't remember him ever performing, but I do remember that he told a story. A story about his trip to Hawaii on a vacation with his brother. He told the story every time I saw him. Every month. For every year that we had Silent Dinners. On his trip he saw palm trees and ate pineapple. He walked on sandy beaches. He flew in a great big plane. He re-lived that adventure once a month with us, and then returned to his farm until the next Silent Dinner.

Those Silent Dinners often run on Deaf Time. Because the Deaf rarely get to hang out with other Deaf, when they do hang out, they have a lot to talk about. What would be a 30-minute lunch for a group of hearing friends is a three-hour affair with the Deaf. When we have Silent Dinners now, we are always closing down the eatery. The staff works around us, sweeping and putting chairs on tables. The conversations of the Deaf not only center around the latest news in someone's life, like marriages and babies, but they also trade information like who got a great deal on a car. Where that great deal was made. And, unlike hearing culture, how much they paid for the car. In our hearing culture, that information would be rude to ask or rude to advertise. But in Deaf culture, it is rude to keep it a secret. Information is important, not a ruler to judge by. If X Car Company will give a Deaf person a fair deal, then the Deaf want to know so that they can go there as well. If Y Car Company worked a shady deal, then the Deaf want to know to avoid it. If a doctor in town is easy to work with in getting an interpreter and patiently working with them until they understand procedures and medications, then the Deaf want to know. That doctor will soon find that she is the most popular doctor in all the land.

In this way, Silent Dinners serve a greater purpose than just hanging out with friends, although the laughter is a big bonus. It is a grand information swap. Language is a lifeline.

The Deaf are 150% more likely to be victims of abuse.
(from the Abused Deaf Women's Advocacy Services [ADWAS]
website #whowillanswer)
At least 50% of Deaf girls are sexually abused
as compared to 25% of hearing girls.
Approximately 54% of deaf boys have been sexually abused as
compared to approximately 10% of hearing boys.
(The National Child Traumatic Stress Network [NCTSN] 2006)

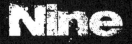

Schools

"There's a sound, a sound, that every heartbeat makes/
It steals through your keyhole till you feel the floorboards
shake/And there is no escaping the rhythm it creates/When
the first downbeat falls." (lines 13-16)
Michael Higgins, "In This House"

In Smalltown, I often found myself in powerless positions under shocking circumstances. One such occasion involved the special education coordinator for the county. I was in her office for different reasons when the topic of my interpreting came up. She told me that the county as a rule would not service Deaf children who needed an interpreter. They advised the family to send the children to the School for the Deaf or move to another county.

I was shocked by her dismissiveness and inquired more.

She said that a number of years before the county had a Deaf child so they hired an interpreter from Alabama who had moved for the job. Soon after the school year began, the family decided to send the Deaf child to the school for the deaf. The interpreter was out of a job. Since that time, the county refused to service Deaf children. (Recent reports support this old policy.) This is a violation of ADA, but the only ones to fight that are the parents themselves.

I went home and asked my Deaf friends, who confirmed the story. I inquired as to why they didn't push the matter because the law was on their side. They ranted about the evil, manipulative hearing world and said there could be no justice. They had grown up in that community as second-class citizens, always being pushed aside, left out, and ignored.

They were never taught their rights, or how to fight for them. Their parents never learned to sign. Who was to teach the children to fight when they never saw it modeled?

The Deaf adults and children who attend a Deaf school speak of it like a true sanctuary where everyone speaks their language, where they can really learn, and be free to be themselves. There they create their own culture, folklore, traditions. They develop a sacred heritage and pride. They defend it fiercely.

A Deaf storyteller and comedian, Peter Cook, has many videos and DVDs where he performs some of the Deaf folklore, many of which began in schools for the deaf. One of those stories is "White Ape" from his video *Terps! And Tales from Deaf Culture* (PC Productions, 2007). The story cannot be done justice simply with these words because the stories are intended to be seen and not heard, but here goes my version in English words.

Once upon a time there were three 11-year-old boys, Jack, John, and Sam, who were always getting into trouble at their residential school for the deaf. They were not bad boys, but they were longing for adventure and a diversion from the long, boring lessons in reading, writing and arithmetic. A rumor had been going around school about a man-eating gorilla that lived on the school grounds. The boys had tried on many occasions to find the gorilla's hiding place, but with no success. One day when Jack was in the principal's office being scolded yet again, he noticed a door hidden in the corner with scrapes on the floor where the door had been opened frequently and with some force. He also noticed bits of banana peel dangling from the handle. He hatched a plan.

That night he and his two friends grabbed their flashlights and pocketknives, and tiptoed down the dark corridors. Sam was the quiet, steady one of the boys. He used the pocketknife and jimmied open the door. John was the scaredy cat who was prone to panic. He was the lookout. Jack was the bold brute and ringleader who liked to tell the others what to do.

As they sneaked into the principal's office, Jack used his flashlight to direct a path to the door he had seen earlier. Sam inspected the doorknob. The banana bits were gone. He gingerly gripped the doorknob and slowly turned it. It followed his direction. Sam had to pull hard to get the door to open. They could feel the vibrations it made on the floor. John started sweating and looked like he could burst into tears.

Jack shined his flashlight into the abyss beyond the door and sure enough, he spotted what he knew had to be the secret passageway to the hidden gorilla. Directly behind that door was a set of steep stairs that descended into some kind of cellar or basement that the boys had never known existed. Jack immediately jumped onto the top step and started running down them. Sam turned to John to allow him to follow next, but John looked as though he might faint. He had turned a gray color. Sam put a hand on his back and pushed him through the door, shutting the office door behind him. They followed Jack's fading light down the stairs.

The bottom of the stairs met a long, cold, damp hallway. Jack waited for the other boys to join him; then John pushed between the two and hooked arms with them. They glanced at each other, and then began the trek down the hallway, side-by-side, arm in arm. The hallway seemed to go on for an eternity. Turn one corner and then another. The light bounced off of the cinder block, gray walls. Eventually they arrived at a metal door with a large steering-wheel-like handle attached. It looked a lot like the doors shown on ships or submarines. The boys instinctively knew that the treasure they sought — the mythical gorilla creature was somewhere behind that door. They were terrified, and yet, they knew that they could never turn back now. No matter what happened.

Jack looked at Sam and nodded then nudged his head toward the door. Sam understood that he was the one to turn the wheel and release the lock while Jack held the light.

Sam could feel the resistance of the old metal wheel turning, but turn it did! One turn. Then another. Finally, on the third turn he felt the lock release, so he slowly pushed the door open into the next room. Jack turned the light back into the black abyss. There it was. Cage bars. The boys were drawn to it as if they were under some magician's spell. They all numbly set one foot in front of the other, first Jack, then Sam, and yes, even John.

Curiosity and boyish sense of adventure were their only instinctive responses. The thought of danger did not enter their minds at the moment of realizing that all of the mythical stories were about to be seen in the flesh. The boys crept closer and closer to the cage, leaving the door behind them wide open. They entered single file until they reached the cage then lined up facing the cage in chorus line fashion. Jack's flashlight circled the 6X6 cage he thought was proving to be empty, when all of a sudden, from the top of the cage dropped an enormous black, furry, red-eyed, yellow-toothed, snarling, angry gorilla that looked like he ate little boys for breakfast. The boys were instantly petrified. Full panic mode froze their feet solidly to the ground so that fight or flight response was of no help – to any of them. The gorilla shook the bars of his cage and roared his large mouth with putrid breath blowing the boys hair back from their faces.

Jack was the first to gain his nerve. He realized that the gorilla could not reach them, so he braved a few steps closer. Sam, emboldened by Jack's clarity of senses, followed and stepped closer. John saw the other two and started shaking his head back and forth, slowly at first then faster.

The gorilla reacted to the two boys' bravado and roared all the more angrily, and shook the bars of the cage all the more violently. His breath became hotter. His eyes became redder. Steam seemed to pour from his ears. Jack wanted to be able to brag that he was brave enough to touch the beast, so he dared a step closer and punched the air between them quickly so as to touch the arm of the gorilla before the beast had the chance to notice what was happening. But Jack did not know of the fast reflexes of a grown, angry gorilla. The gorilla answered his action with a darting hand of his own, whose human-like hand grabbed Jack's wrist before he his reflexes could jerk his hand back. The gorilla wrapped his hand around Jack's wrist and pulled him to the cage. Sam leapt to Jack to pull him back. John melted into hysteria. The gorilla reached his other arm through the cage, dove his wrinkled fingers at Jack's face, and pinched his nose.

The gorilla released the boy, took a step back and seemed to laugh at him. The boys didn't have time to mentally register what had just happened. They fell to the floor when the gorilla released Jack. Sam had stumbled, but not fallen to the ground. He grabbed Jack by the scruff of the neck, grabbed John by the arm, and drug both of them backwards through the open metal door. He didn't bother closing it behind him. The other two boys gained their feet and the three of them sprinted back down the hallway, running faster than they ever had in their whole lives. They darted up the stairs, slammed the door closed, and rushed out of the principal's office, not bothering to be sneaky and unnoticed.

That night in their beds, the boys swore to themselves that from that day on they would be good boys and never break rules again.

The gorilla returned to his corner to eat a banana, fully pleased wit the night's events.

In recent years, some states have adopted a Deaf Child Bill of Rights that focuses on the specific needs of Deaf children, a population grossly neglected in many places. Many Deaf children enter kindergarten not having any language. Some don't know their own names. While they are learning to express their basic needs and wants, they are expected to learn and retain content in science and social studies. Benchmark tests add unfair disadvantage by asking questions using Dr. Seuss nonsense words or questions about music or common knowledge questions that would not be common knowledge to a Deaf child: 3 little pigs, 3 bears. The Deaf culture has its own folklore but a Deaf child in a hearing family would not know either set of stories.

Recent legislation in some states has helped with much of the language problem by requiring early hearing testing so that early intervention allows the children to receive language of some kind at an earlier age.

In some states, American Sign Language (ASL) is acknowledged as a foreign language. In some it is not; therefore, Deaf students who want to go to college must take French, Spanish, Chinese or German (which have spoken components) in order to qualify for college. Their knowledge of ASL and English should qualify as two languages. Many Deaf are very skilled in other languages, but for so many it is an unreasonable and unnecessary challenge that can keep many deserving students from college.

I once met parents of a deaf 12-year-old girl who were fighting the school system over services for the child. The young lady had endured many surgeries to "fix" her deafness. Her parents refused to allow her to sign for fear she would never try to speak. They would not allow the Deaf man who was the deaf educator to work with her on reading because the teacher's speech was not clear. The result was a 12-year-old girl who could not read, speak, or sign. She did not have Deaf friends or hearing friends because she could not communicate with either. The parents' efforts to make their daughter "normal" served to make her isolated in a sea of children.

A Deaf little boy was participating in the grade-level musical, the teachers asked the child to mouth the words like the other children. I suggested the hand movements could easily be changed from dance moves to signs and be understandable by the Deaf child, teach sign to all of the children, and retain the musicality of the production. The music teacher did that for one song. The other 19 songs were danced and mouthed.

There was a huge glimmer of hope for this child, however, in the form of his classroom teacher. The classroom teacher of that child learned sign language and even taught the students throughout the year: alphabet, numbers, reading vocabulary, and signs for different places in the school. By the end of the year, the students and their teacher basically communicated with the Deaf student free of an interpreter.

One day in the library, near the end of the school year, the librarian came to me and said, "These kids have learned a lot of sign language this year!"

I had to step step back and notice for the first time. The children were walking up to the Deaf child and asking to trade crayons or books and asking to sit with him—all in his language. He was like a celebrity. It was beautiful. It was as it should be. It was an example of how things could be if we adults would allow a natural chain of events to happen and not try to fix what we see as broken.

This experience was a teachable moment for me as well. I saw what effect the right people in the right places doing the right things can do. Even though many other situations in the school were inappropriate and counter-productive, one person doing the right thing made a big impact, not only on the education of the child, but also on the self-esteem of the child. For the first time, I felt that I had witnessed how a Deaf child could grow up in a hearing family with hearing teachers in a hearing environment and still be wholly educated and feel valued.

That to me was the modern day example of the Martha's Vineyard model of what was to become the Sign Club Co. (Story page 122).

"…to my list'ning ears / All nature sings, and round me rings The music of the spheres." (verse 1)
Maltbie D. Babcock, 1901, "This Is My Father's World"

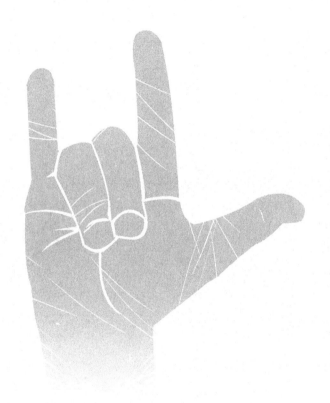

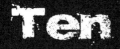

Ten

Bob's Daughter's Surgery

"Have you spoken a word full of hope and cheer? Have you walked with a slower pace, Till the weary of heart who were stumbling on, Took new Courage to / run the race?" (verse 2)

Lizzie DeArmond, 1916, "O the Things We May Do"

My Deaf friend Bob had a daughter who needed surgery to remove metal plates from a previously broken arm. I went with them to sit in the waiting room. We talked; I sewed; we planned parties and solved the world's problems. When the surgery was over, the young surgeon came to the waiting room and asked me to sit with the young lady in recovery until she woke-up. Bob agreed, so I went.

On the walk back to the recovery room, the doctor said to me, "You need to tell them (the Deaf family) to find out what is wrong with their genetics so that it can be fixed. Three generations of deafness must be heredity, so they need to find a way to fix it before it happens again."

I don't know what my face said, but in my head my mouth was dropping in disbelief. This wasn't a doctor from the Middle Ages. He was young. Not long out of medical school. How could he hold such archaic beliefs? 'What is wrong with them?!' 'Fix it?!' I had read about that philosophy, but I had never experienced it until that moment.

Fifteen years have passed since then. Unfortunately, I have learned that the doctor's views are more prevalent than I could ever believe. The Deaf world has words to explain it, but they all revolve around a hearing world's reluctance to accept deafness as an option. To accept that there is an alternative reality. To be deaf does not mean one has to be disabled. To be deaf does not mean one has to have surgeries and be dependent on hearing technology.

Is it an option? YES! It is a viable solution for many.

Is it required for a quality life? NO!

I have many Deaf friends who have cochlear implants or hearing aids and are perfectly happy. I also have many Deaf friends who are profoundly deaf and do not ever want to have cochlear implants or hearing aids because they are completely happy. Shockingly for the hearing world, I have many deaf friends who have grown into adulthood and removed their cochlear implants and hearing aids because they were not happy. The hearing world doesn't understand. For a hearing person to become deaf would be a tragedy because we are dependent on our ears for communicating. There is, however, an alternative reality that is free from wearing technology that fails, breaks, and is expensive.

I have seen this line drawn in the sand all of my life. This war between the oral deaf and the signing Deaf. I have friends in both arenas and I love them all. I don't choose a side. I choose to accept each person for who he is and what he has chosen for himself. Professionally, I find that I am an advocate for the Deaf children who sign simply because those Deaf have fewer people who are advocating for them. I grew up in the Deaf World of signing, highly literate, gainfully employed, and for the most part, functioning families of people. They lived before cochlear implants and they were very happy with a quality life. The warring arenas only serve to dissuade potential allies in the fight for equality and suppress the potential of future generations of deaf children. Instead of drawing lines of differences between us, we need to be drawing circles that draw us together. We all have something in common. We should build on the ways we are alike and learn from the ways we are different. We all have greater enemies of cancer and AIDS and poverty and abuse. If we can focus on those challenges, fight those enemies instead of each other, we would find that the world is a place of music and harmony after all.

Personally, I will admit, when I am in a noisy hotel trying to sleep, that I am envious of the deaf who can sleep in silent bliss through the noisiest rock band next door.

Compare that doctor's view to the Deaf view. I once met a Deaf gentleman who was the thirteenth-generation Deaf. It was like a pedigree. He was a blueblood. His son was the first generation born hearing. It was a tragedy in his family. Why? Because the family culture was broken. The heritage lost.

No longer could father and son share experiences from the school for the deaf or deaf movies. What about the football game when Steven Tyler sang the National Anthem? That experience was not the same for father and son even though the outcome of the game was the same. Life happened in two different worlds forever more. I would love to have introduced the thirteenth-generation Deaf man to the young surgeon. I bet sparks would have flown. Their clash of cultures would have brought more education than all of those years of chemistry ever could.

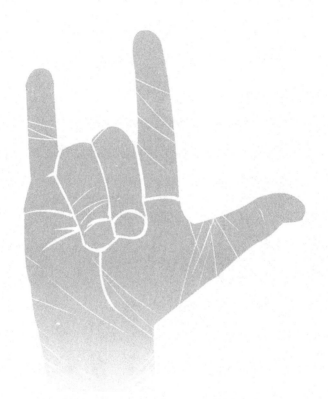

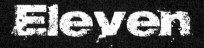

Eleven

Interpreter School
"All the music needs is a place to begin
In this house that we're all living in." (lines 31-32)
Michael Higgins, "In This House"

I actually met the thirteenth-generation Deaf man while I was taking a graduate class. Two friends and I made it to the two-week class where thirteenth-generation man was an instructor. In the class were about fifteen more interpreters from around the country.

This is where my first experience in interpreter pecking order began. When interpreters (and some Deaf) learn that I was introduced to the Deaf world through church, their response is invariably an "Oh, that," with their noses in the air and a look on their faces like I just admitted to eating paste. I am very aware that many people in church will copy signs from a book or internet, teach a group of kids, and call themselves interpreters, never having met or signed with an actual Deaf person. People who hire interpreters very often don't know how to hire an interpreter and will hire anyone who wiggles their hands with confidence.

The Registry of Interpreters for the Deaf (RID) has set standards and legitimized the profession, but for many of us in rural, backwoods trenches, we don't have the luxury of a Deaf Enforcer. We see the Deaf go without access...anywhere. We are powerless to do anything about it. In many places, I found my role was often the link between the hearing world and the Deaf world. And my Deaf world experience began in Deaf church. It had many characteristics to a CODA's experience, only I learned church vocabulary instead of slang and profanity. I had to take a class to learn to cuss in sign.

When I returned home from the two-week graduate class and talked with the Center on Deafness's Boss Lady, I said, "I don't need to be an interpreter. The class taught me that I know nothing."

Boss Lady said, "Did you struggle understanding the Deaf?"

"No," I said. "I understood the Deaf teachers, but the other interpreters from around the country—some I couldn't understand at all. I don't have the training or education or certifications that they do."

She said, "As long as you and the Deaf communicate well, don't worry about the rest."

I have survived on that phrase for many years.

At that two-week workshop, I found some other experiences useful. During a weekend immersion, we were not allowed to speak with our voices or use our hearing for communication: telephones (before texting), alarm clocks. We could only use visual aids: TTY, flashing alarm clocks, or friends who would tap us awake.

That weekend in the country included a neighbor who spun out on the gravel road where the house sat. We were awake all night listening. The Deaf slept soundly and laughed at our droopy eyes the next morning. While shopping for groceries, we heard people's comments and frustrations because of our "deafness."

There was a Deaf 18-month-old child there with his Deaf parents at our immersion. As we were outside, he ran toward the road while a car was coming. I realized yelling at him was useless. We had to chase him and get in front of him. I thought of all the stresses with children and felt overwhelmed by the added responsibilities of parents with Deaf children.

Of course, that 18-month-old also had a large vocabulary since both of his parents were Deaf. Because I had not been around many Deaf babies, especially those with Deaf parents, I was thrilled to see how a Deaf child who is exposed to language early can develop as normally as any child. The 18-month-old would sign C-A-R for his toy car. He couldn't distinguish a 'C' or 'A' or 'R,' but he knew those hand shapes represented the toy he loved. This was very impressive, and set the stage for reading readiness. Young hearing children also know that the spoken word "car" represents their beloved toy, but cannot yet distinguish the letters that make the word.

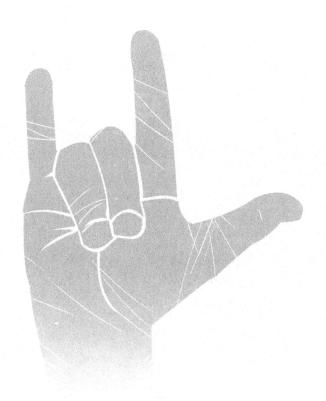

Twelve

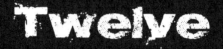

Cussing Class

"Good mornin' life…here we are/One more day…what's in
the cards?/Doesn't matter anyway, I'm gonna have to play/
The hand you give me." (lines 1-4)

Larry Haack and Michael Higgins, "The Song You Give Me"

I had heard rumors of a child in the county who was notorious for sexual, indecent behavior. I had heard other interpreters talking about the history and escapades of the child. I was terrified of having to sub for that assignment. My experiences so far in the Deaf world were based in church; therefore, I had never learned how to cuss or how to explain various sexual terms, positions, and deviations. I was scared. Since I was required to have 20 hours of professional development, I looked for a workshop on how to do just that.

I found a workshop about 10 hours away. It was an all day workshop on a Saturday. A lady who had been an educational interpreter for many years in a school system that had an excellent Deaf Ed. program taught the workshop.

The interpreter's job is to say (or sign) everything that is said in conversation or the classroom. No filters. No inhibitions. Faithfully interpret. So if a seventeen-year-old boy is talking about what he did on Friday night, the interpreter is signing it. If the Deaf student is cussing in sign, the interpreter is voicing it as faithfully and authentically as possible. Ideally, everyone forgets that the student is Deaf and that the interpreter is present.

This opens up a whole other world of problems for interpreters in school systems. Sometimes interpreters are punished for cussing. Sometimes the Deaf student is not punished because he is a 'poor little deaf kid'.

This is where the workshop began. It was held near a college with an interpreter training program (ITP), so there were a lot of college students participating. They dominated the interactive portion when we had to give English terms and descriptions of various sexual positions and sexual games. My heart went out to all of the little old ladies in the room who looked like they were having a difficult time. They had probably been introduced to interpreting just like I had – in church.

The first six hours of the workshop involved us being told that if we had problems with any of the sex or vulgar language, we were in the wrong profession. I was screaming on the inside, "THAT IS WHAT I HAVE BEEN SAYING!"

And that is what I took away from the workshop. All the way home I tried to scour my head of all of the images that we had been talking about how to interpret. I just prayed I would never have to use them.

I actually learned from my adult deaf friends. I sat one down one day and asked him to teach me to cuss. He laughed, but agreed. Of course, he cussed like an old guy. He didn't know the new cuss words. It got me started anyway. When I got to the middle school and high school, they taught me the rest. And when the students learn that the interpreters are catching on to the curse words, they change them.

Awkwardly, I learned some foreign curse words, too. Once I was speaking to a group of business leaders in the community, and I taught them what I have found to be the most important sign in sign language – bathroom. It is the letter "T" in sign language (you know, like when you are little and someone says, "I've got your nose!" with their thumb tucked between the first two fingers?), shaken back and forth. (You will see other signs for restroom, but this is the one most frequently used in our corner of the country). I noticed that when I showed the sign, a gasp came from somewhere on my left. No one seemed to be in medical need so I went on with the speech. When it was all over, a Korean gentleman came up to me and said that in Korean sign language, that sign was the equivalent of "shooting the bird" in American culture. I hee-hawed laughing, thinking what a funny moment that had to be for that poor gentleman. But now I know to never sign that in Korea.

The cussing and vulgarity I was eventually called upon to use. I interpreted as faithfully as possible without filters. Then wrestled with my conscience all the way home. I knew that the words didn't originate with me, yet the words came from my mouth...or hands. I could only picture the disappointed faces of all of my Sunday School teachers. But the inner turmoil didn't stop there. Like many Southern girls, I wilt at the first sign of conflict, yet this journey is nothing but.

I have heard of a story that a distinguished history museum

wanted to present a Deaf exhibit and contacted a Deaf organization to coordinate it. An oral deaf group heard about it and became upset because they, too, were deaf and should be included. The two groups fought until the museum decided not to hold the exhibit after all.

I have heard on numerous occasions arguments, disagreements, and debates on which signing system is best to teach deaf children: Signed Exact English, American Sign Language, Contact, PSE, Cued speech, etc.

I have heard numerous arguments about whether or not a Deaf child should be given an interpreter at all since they will have to learn to live independently eventually.

I have heard MANY arguments and debates about cochlear implants versus signing...

Certified versus Qualified interpreters
Deaf schools versus Mainstreamed
Zoned schools versus Bused to one location, central schools
Certified interpreters versus Higher taxes
Deaf versus Hearing

The arguments go on and on and on, and yet we just celebrated 25 years of ADA. Clearly, we have work still to do, because 25 years of ADA have not yet reached the corners of rural America. Children (and adults) are still denied access to communication in too many schools and courts- the very places where there should be equality.

The truth is that for every line drawn in division a fracture is created in the fragile ground we gain. The arguing is divisive and self-defeating. The arguing creates chaos. We can each have different points of view. That is okay, good even. Like with music, different sounds can blend together for an even better effect. It is called harmony. What we need is harmony. Each part blending with other parts to weave beautiful music. If we were creating beautiful "music," we would find more "singers" and "listeners."

We must learn to work together to create harmony. Find

common ground. Work toward the same goals. Build on each other's strengths. Fight common enemies, not each other.

Angry words! O let them never From the tongue unbridled slip;
May the heart's best impulse ever Check them ere they soil the lip.
'Love one another'….
Love is much too pure and holy, Friendship is too sacred far,
For a moment's reckless folly Thus to desolate and mar.
'Love one another'….
Angry words are lightly spoken, Bitt'rest tho'ts are rashly stirred,
Brightest links of life are broken By a single angry word.
'Love one another'…. (verses 1-3)
Sunday School Teacher, 1867, "Angry Words"

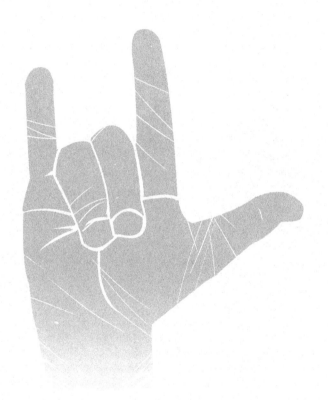

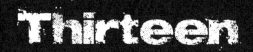

Thirteen

A.D.A. Meeting

"…Whenever clouds arise,
When song gives place to sighing, When hope within me
dies…." (verse 3)

Civilla D. Martin, 1906, "His Eye Is on the Sparrow"

A big OMG moment for me was in Smalltown when we set-up a meeting with the county officials to discuss A.D.A. I used money we had raised to pay for an interpreter, buy sign language books for the police department and pay for an education for Bobby's wife to become the first interpreter in the county.

For our meeting, the Deaf baked brownies, the church bought punch, and I sent formal invitations to the County Executive, City Manager, Chief of Police and Fire, Sheriff, Special Education Coordinator and many other officials in the county. We also invited an A.D.A. specialist from Big Town to speak.

I had called an A.D.A. specialist attorney to come as well. While on the phone, he asked, "So tell me, what exactly does the A.D.A. say about interpreters?" …Oh, boy. I didn't ask him to come after all.

The day of the meeting arrived. Showtime. - The speaker showed up an hour late…and, I think, drunk.

It didn't matter anyway. No one came.

It taught me quite a few things. Primarily, it taught me why the 'state of things was so rotten' for the Deaf. It taught me that those in positions of authority do not hold the best interest of those with disabilities. In fact, those who are supposed to be allies are doing more damage than good. It also taught me that unless the Deaf do it themselves, take up arms and defend their own rights, nothing would change.

The reaction of the Deaf that day was that of any other day. They were not surprised. It was as it always had been for them.

My reaction was frustration with myself that I had been so naïve, anger that the powers that be were so apathetic, and exhausted at the thought of all the work to be done.

I realized that if anything were to change, something much bigger than me was going to have to do it. I just didn't know who or what that was.

Bubba

"People talking without speaking.
People hearing without listening./
People writing songs that voices never share..." (lines 17-19)
Simon and Garfunkel, "The Sounds of Silence"

The most significant lesson for me up to that point was an upcoming trial, which involved a Deaf friend of mine. He had tested positive for the HIV virus. The woman who had passed the virus to him had knowingly slept with him and fifty-one others without informing them of the risk or offering protection. This was the first case of its kind in the world, so all major news networks would be parked on the courthouse lawn. My friend was the only person of the fifty-two at that point to test positive for the virus. He was scheduled to be a witness and testify on the stand.

The attorney called me and said she wanted me to interpret.

I replied, "No. I can't. I am so not qualified. For this assignment, you need a court certified interpreter."

"I'll pay you $100," she said.

"It's not about the money. Anything I interpret can be thrown out of court. I am not trained to do what you are asking. I can give you the phone number for a group of interpreters who are qualified to do this."

"If you won't do it, then we just won't have an interpreter," she affirmed.

I called the Deaf Center again.

"Boss Lady, what do I do?!" I asked. "Bubba can't go on the stand without someone to interpret. Isn't it law that they must provide an interpreter?"

"No," she replied. "The law requires the defendant to have an interpreter. Don't worry. I'll be there. I will show them how it works and should be done."

She did come. And she interpreted for twelve hours—for free. I sat in the audience and interpreted proceedings for the Deaf who had come, but Boss Lady interpreted actual court proceedings. I was so grateful.

The police and investigators had used pen and paper to question Bubba. This had the potential of being thrown out of court because it was not reliable information. Nationally, the deaf graduate with about a third to fourth-grade reading level. Some don't read at all. They don't read newspapers, which are usually written at about an eighth grade reading level. Think about it like most of hearing English speakers who take two years of a foreign language in high school. If we were taken to Mexico or France, we could not communicate at the same level as the natives of the country in their language.

That misunderstanding of cultures came up in the trial. While Bubba was on the stand, the defense attorney cross-examined him saying, "Do you really expect us to believe you have never heard of the HIV virus? Have you never watched the news report or read the newspaper? You expect us to believe that?"

I was in the audience about to run a blitz on the court proceedings. I wanted to stamp my foot and give that attorney a piece of my mind. Yes, it is very possible that every bit of what that attorney said was true! How dare he be so insulting and condescending!

I didn't rush the stand, though, and I was very, very grateful that Boss Lady was there. Unlike my inclinations, she was very professional.

Late that night, when the trial was over, CNN wanted an interview with Bubba. Boss Lady interpreted. Thank God for that, too.

50% of 18-year-old deaf and hard of hearing students read below fourth grade level compared to 1% of their hearing peers. (Traxler, 2000)

Fourteen

Move to Bigger Town

"…Bring in the day of brotherhood And end the night of wrong." (verse 2)

William P. Merrill, 1911, "Rise Up, O Men of God"

After the leadership at the Smalltown church asked the Deaf preacher to leave his pulpit, the Deaf World concluded that the church hated Deaf people. To this day a Deaf person has not darkened its doorway.

I knew the Deaf in the area needed a church home. Fortunately, I also knew a gentleman in a nearby town who worked as the educational minister at his local congregation whose numbers could accommodate a Deaf group. I also knew that he had knowledge of the church where I had grown up and would be closer to understanding the Deaf than anyone else around.

I drove to Bigger Town and knocked on his door. He set-up a meeting with the leadership and within a week we started interpreting services and teaching sign classes. Forty people came to the classes including every member of the leadership. Eight people stuck it out and started interpreting. In about 18 months, I turned it all over to them and returned to my family and the church in Smalltown. The church in Bigger Town is still the home for the Deaf in the area.

Soon afterward, we moved to Big City and I had every intention of leaving the Deaf behind.

Jonah ran from Nineveh, too.

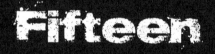

My First Big City Assignment

"So he spends his nights down in the trenches/With the
keepers of the alleyways and the park benches." (lines 17-18)
Michael Higgins and Jeb Stuart Anderson, "Love Ain't Everything"

When we moved to Big City, I had my full-time job within my field of study. I was ready to be a professional and forget the ugliness and prickliness of the Deaf World, which continually drained me of all positivity and energy. I had fought battles that were not mine to fight. I had been taken advantage of by every facet of society. I had wept many a tear over this dysfunctional relationship with the Deaf World and wanted no more to do with it. I also knew Big City because I had grown up with it. I knew I wasn't the kind of interpreter Big City wanted. I was not pedigreed.

I was a teacher of English. The principal at the school where I worked had told me that I needed to sponsor a club. I knew the appeal that sign language had for kids, so I sponsored a Sign Club. It was a big hit. We only met a few times during the year, but the girls—almost always is—were excited and eager.

After two years there, the Deaf community had again been calling. The needs are great. The workers are few. I signed up with the Deaf Center as a freelance interpreter. My intention was to take assignments that other, more qualified, interpreters could not take. I was the "whenever you are desperate" interpreter; a warm body.

My first assignment was at a hospital. Just to sit with the Deaf man in recovery until he woke-up and was moved to his room. Simple.

Because this was Big City, I was prepping myself to be professional in the extreme. Expectations were higher. Clients were highly educated. High stakes. Pedigrees. Bluebloods. I put on the appropriate clothing and mask, ready for a refreshing difference from Smalltown.

When I arrived to relieve the other interpreter, the gentleman was actually awake. I walked to the side of the bed to introduce myself. A nurse stood on his opposite side, attending to nurse-like duties.

The Deaf man immediately signed to me, "F-A-R-T me."

I blinked. I blinked again. Surely, I had misunderstood. Surely, he didn't just sign what I thought he had.

"Again, please," I signed.

"F-A-R-T me," he repeated.

I stared blankly. The nurse asked, "What did he say?"

I mechanically turned my head to look at her and said, "I think he is telling us he needs to fart."

I looked back at him, and he nodded his head in question, asking if I had interpreted for him.

I nodded back.

He then leaned on his side towards me, lifted the sheet, and set off what sounded like a foghorn.

I couldn't believe it. I turned my back to him quickly to control my need to laugh hysterically and squelch tears of disillusionment.

As I turned back, the nurse was looking at me with a look of exasperation and said, "Well, at least he warned us."

My dreams of leaving the battles and frustrations of the Deaf World behind me blew up cruelly and toxically in those fumes. I had not escaped after all.

Richard

"As long as I'm breathin' and I can see that light/I'm gonna be reachin' for that highest high/I'll keep believin' and keep singin'..."
(lines 9-12)
Larry Haack and Michael Higgins, "The Song You Give Me"

The Deaf world came back, bigger than ever. I clearly wasn't getting the message. In Big City my family began attending a church of 1500 people. Within a few months, we met a man who was Deaf and had been a member there for over 30 years with no interpreter.

And so it began again.

I started interpreting for him and together we started sign language classes. I thought, "In congregations of 350+ in other churches, 40 people came to classes. Eight stuck with me each time. Surely, here with 1500 we'll have a great turnout." Thirteen people came. None interpreted.

Richard told me that for 30 years he sat in the back of the auditorium and cried and asked God to help him. So, when I started feeling sorry for myself, I thought of him and decided I had many years of patience ahead of me before I got to Richard's level.

Richard had grown up during a time and place when signing was frowned upon. Parents were told not to teach their children to sign. That is still a philosophy around the area now, but many families have migrated in who are from parts of the country where American Sign Language (ASL) is king and the Deaf world is bold and strong.

Richard's growing up years are a wonder to me. He does wear hearing aids, and he is one of the best lip readers I have ever met. However, the "average deaf adult with years of speechreading practice does not read lips much better than the average hearing adult" (Marschark 15). If you think about how often teachers speak while writing on the board and looking down into a book, or how often students around the classroom will be engaged in a debate with rapid fire and no indication from whence the next statement may come...how in the world Richard survived high school amazes me.

He learned sign language the summer after high school graduation when he went to Gallaudet University. All classes are taught in ASL, so he had to learn—and fast. He is now a photographer on the side. The photography company where he worked would not allow him to actually take pictures. They even refused him interpreters during staff meetings and refused visual fire alarms for safety. He did pursue the matter with a disability/legal aid agency, but they needed him to drive two hours to meet with them during the work day...taking time off to sue the company you work for isn't good business. So he dropped it. When he does have time off, he takes amazing photos of still life and events like the Fourth of July festival fireworks. Every time we have an event, we call him.

The interpreting at Big Town church is different from the other churches because I am the only interpreter. In the past I had a team of people to share hymns, sermons, and then Sunday morning service, Sunday night service, and church events like potlucks and fall carnivals. At Big Town, it was only me.

Ideally, an interpreter will have access to the information ahead of time: sermon topic, scripture readings, hymns for service. The parts that can be prepared ahead of time should be. Hymns, for example, are sometimes written 200 years ago and written in Old English. The words must be translated from Old English into modern English and then into ASL. One of the hardest hymns I have found to translate is "The Church's One Foundation." One of the phrases in the hymn is "the charter of salvation." I can remember sitting on my bed with half-a-dozen books and dictionaries scattered across the bed, my husband in a chair with paper and pen, as we tried to decide what the sentence was really saying and how to put that into visual understanding that could be signed musically in the space of time that the hearing congregation would be singing it—hours of work.

The lecturers become easier to interpret with time, usually. If an interpreter works with the same speaker for a period of time, the interpreter begins to acquire the speaker's voice. However, guest speakers, especially specialists in their fields, are some of the hardest to interpret for because they use a specialized vocabulary that the interpreter may not be familiar with. I find the hardest speakers are the ones who tell preacher stories because I can't predict the outcome. I frequently will leave out pertinent information simply because I didn't know it was pertinent at the time. Or the punchline is funny only to a hearing audience. It is a play on words or accents, totally lost to a deaf crowd. The deaf look around at the hearing who are laughing and look at me wondering why they aren't. I shrug and say, 'I am sorry. Dumb hearing joke.' Then move on.

One of the funniest interpreting moments was when a guest speaker from Scotland took the pulpit. He was telling stories about what I thought were poppies in a field. After quite a few confusing minutes of story, I realized it was not poppies but puppies. Then I was laughing hysterically, and no one else was. The deaf were truly confused.

We live and learn.

Of the thirteen people who came to sign language classes at the 1500-size church, one was a parent of a deaf lady and one was deaf. Both had been a part of the time period of Richard when signing was forbidden. Teaching sign language to a deaf person is a humbling experience; an experience I feel immeasurably unqualified for, but I did the best I could. Most of the people in the class were intrigued by the language and thought it was beautiful. Even though they did not want to help interpret, they did become a family for Richard and provided him with connections at the church that he had not had before.

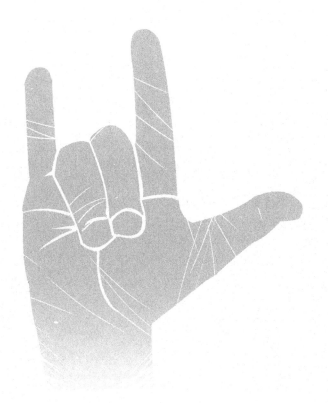

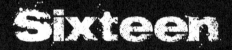

The Children

"In this house, there are many doors/And mine is right next to yours/The space that separates us is very thin/In this house that we are living in." (lines 21-24)

Michael Higgins, "In This House"

I thought I knew the Deaf World well. I had grown up in it. I had worked in it as a friend and volunteer. I had never been a professional in it until the day I went into the schools. I began a lesson then that rocked my world. I had never witnessed the world from their perspective until then. These are their stories as told by an army of interpreters or by the children themselves.

Can you count the birds that warble In the sunshine all the day?
Can you count the little fishes That in sparkling waters play?...
Can you count the many children In their little beds at night,
Who without a thought of sorrow Rise again at morning light?...
(verses 2-3)
Johann Hey, 1837, and Tr., Elmer L. Jorgenson, 1921,
"Can You Count the Stars?"

Franco

I was brought onto the interpreting staff in the local public school for one particular little boy who had just moved into the community. He was in preschool and he was as cute as a chow puppy. He had chubby little cheeks and great big eyes that exposed childlike curiosity and deep-seeded distrust and frustration. He had minimal signs. The ones he did know were animal signs. That is not helpful for explaining one's feelings or communicating basic needs like 'I am hungry' and 'I need to go to the bathroom'. He was notorious for a temper and stubborn streak. For those who work with children who have problems communicating, that is not surprising.

Franco, however, was brilliant. I watched him stand in a chair and study the caterpillars in their little tent hoping to see them turn into butterflies. Every morning, Franco stood in a chair and stared at the fuzzy worms climb and build cocoons and, eventually, morph into flying insects. Franco's little hands copied the wings of the butterfly. He could mimic exactly the flutter or the stretch or the whisper of the wings. I watched him throughout the day stop people in the hallways to explain to them the worm crawling and building and hanging and breaking free to flight. I was amazed every time, and became somewhat addicted to the feeling of awe from this brilliant mind. Of course, then the communication breakdown would happen and inevitably, the temper tantrum, and I quickly forgot why I was there at all.

73

I had six weeks with Franco before summer. We had a shaky relationship. He was angry with me, I think, because I was always around him. He had obviously never had experience with an interpreter before, so he didn't realize that I was communicating in his language what everyone else around was saying.

One day as the class was discussing the weather outside, he signed to me that it was sunny. I voiced, "It is sunny." The child whose job was to report on the weather said that it was cloudy. Franco's face instantly turned red and hard when I signed that it was cloudy. He was angry with me and wouldn't look at me for a long time because he thought that I was the one who disagreed with him.

I met his mother and we became friends. I wanted to meet with them over the summer so that when the school year started, Franco and I wouldn't be starting from scratch. I learned from his mom that even though Franco gave me a hard time at school, he talked about me at home. That was hopeful.

I remember Franco getting so excited about the bus. He could only sign "bus." He couldn't tell me what the kids were wearing on the bus, what he saw out the window, what the candy tasted like that the bus drivers gave him. I thought back to when my girls were in preschool. I couldn't get them to stop talking about what had happened at school; endless monologues on food and books and playground equipment. It made me feel desperate to feed the child language—and fast. He was learning, a lot, but he was about to have to start learning content about science, social studies, math and writing. He is one of the very blessed because his family was trying to speak to him in sign language, only they were just learning, too. He needed more. I just didn't know how to get it to him.

Franco's mother, who had come from a state where the Deaf world is much different from Smalltown, was shocked by the archaic philosophy and education of Deaf children. She was appalled that ASL was not accepted as a second language. She was young and willing to fight for Franco's rights. I knew I had found an ally. I wasn't sure how it would end up, but I wanted this relationship to grow.

Why is it that so often, the people who are in charge and making decisions do not have any knowledge or experience in the area in which they are in charge? The movie *Heartbreak Ridge* with

Clint Eastwood is what I often think of as I hear the stories of interpreters in schools. Clint Eastwood's character was a seasoned veteran sergeant who had seen combat in different continents and in different decades, but he wasn't in charge. A young lieutenant fresh from college, who had never seen a battlefield, was calling all of the shots and had the lives of young marines in his hands.

I know that this situation is prevalent in many places, but never had I experienced it so poignantly than when watching Franco—and others like him—suffer because those making decisions about his education had never met a deaf person or studied anything about education for those deaf.

In some school systems, all of the deaf in the county are bussed to one group of schools so that the students can share resources like a team of interpreters and have an environment with other deaf children. Other systems allow the students to attend their zoned schools so that they are closer to home. However, that means that the students may never see another deaf person for all of the years they are in school. They may have access to a deaf education teacher a few times a week. Other than that, their interpreter is their only source of communication, and that interpreter is required to sign only what is communicated for curriculum standards.

Albert

Full of potential, drive, ambition, and zest for life is what ideally every teacher and administrator wants to see in his or her students, especially if the student has an added disadvantage like deafness. Deafness doesn't have to be a disability, and for some it is not. It is merely a speed bump. Albert is one of those kids.

Albert grew up in an inner city home, but with a mom and aunties that drilled Bible verses in his head, and hard work into his core. The family didn't sign, but they communicated the best they could orally with Albert, and they were tight.

Albert was in advanced trig, honors chemistry, and AP History, while his deaf friends were taking Art 101 and goofing-off in gym. Albert had plans to go to college and major in nursing. He paid little attention to the interpreter during class, but instead intently studied the board and looked like he was trying to paint a mental picture in his brain for future retrieval. The only time the student really seemed to pay attention to the interpreter was during down time in class when the interpreter became his playmate and friend.

After school Albert worked a full-time job at the local foodbank. He was saving money to buy a car so that he could get back and forth to college. The college he wanted to attend had a great support system for students with disabilities, but Albert wouldn't be able to afford to live on campus.

He was a success story—the kind that gives hope to those working with these kids.

Kevin

One of Albert's cohorts was equally as smart, but with a different home life. Kevin's home wasn't abusive in the normal sense, but crippling in that it was patronizing and smothering. The family made sure the child knew he was disabled: not able to do anything by himself or make wise decisions on his own. Everything was done for him because he couldn't. This student won a scholarship to Gallaudet, but was told what to major in and told what extra-curricular activities were allowed. Then when young ladies came into the picture, Kevin was told who he could and could not date. Since Kevin had grown up under such control, he accepted what momma said and did as he was told.

Lolita

Her blank eyes tore pity from your soul. Her behaviors would mortify you. She was schizophrenic. She had been sexually abused. She was Deaf and she was mainstreamed.

She was typically oblivious of her surroundings, save sparkly things and paranoid, crazed obsession with imagined sightings of the word "bitch" signed by numerous people in hallways.

As I observed her behaviors all day and she haunted my thoughts all night, I saw the same blank stares in my dog at home. Upon noticing that similarity, I began noticing others.

For example, my dog had a fondness for flipping the trashcan and destroying its contents all over the house. He knew he would be punished for it when I returned home and saw him huddled in a corner instead of barking and jumping at my waist. He knew it was wrong, yet he couldn't seem to stop himself from the offense.

Lolita was the same. Not with trashcans but with baby toys. She hoarded baby toys in her purse, backpack and pockets. She thieved like a magpie and snuck school-illegal contraband: gum and dumdums. Her efforts at sneaking were like those of a two-year-old. She sat wide-eyed, facing me as I interpreted and slowly eased a dumdum from her bag to her mouth, hiding her mouth behind a cupped hand—never blinking, never breaking eye contact.

I had heard stories about Lolita. She was the daughter of a drug addict. The mother pimped out her daughter for money to supply her addiction. The child was removed from the home. While with the custodial family, Lolita was again exposed to more sexual abuse by visiting family and friends. She had a history of sexual acting out all through elementary school.

Lolita had a boyfriend. He also had special needs and was mainstreamed and Lolita was obsessed with him. She had a picture of him that she had torn out of a yearbook. She carried it in her pocket. She talked about him, made up stories about him, drew pictures of him. When Lolita was asked how old he was, she said, "7th." When asked how many years, she said, "I don't know. 5?"

One day a custodian found a note in the hallway with the students' names on it, and she was shocked. Lolita had written to the boyfriend two weeks earlier. The letter contained pictures on the front and back of the paper of oral sex. The pictures of the boy and girl involved in oral sex were quite detailed and anatomically accurate. The school counselor and the social worker were called in. No interpreter was called in to help interview the student.

The next day I met her in class and she seemed to be talking to someone when I entered the room. Actually talking with her mouth. There was no one around her. She did have a cochlear implant, but she could not recognize her name if someone yelled it. She had never been trained to recognize sounds or trained in speech. I had never been quite sure why she was forced to wear it. She actually hated it and frequently cried because it made her head hurt. I had never seen her benefit from any sound that she may have gotten from it.

After lunch one day in the hallway, she told me that she pretended she was a cat and hissed and clawed at her friends in the hall. It explained why the students were giving her funny looks. Lolita then told me that she loved me and we were sisters.

Afterwards she was very upset with me because when she asked me what color her eye shadow was I said blue. She sign-screamed, "It is silver!!"

One time on a bright-blue-eye-shadow-day, she stared at a young man through class. She told me that she couldn't read anymore. Then she said, "Monkey. Scratch bottom. Poops. Funny me say that."

She was mainstreamed in all of her classes except for English. Most days she didn't know where her next class was. A few days she couldn't recognize her own name.

I was told by past interpreters that once upon a time she had been like every other student in the class, and then something happened that sent her spiraling into her current hot mess.

One day her guardian came into the office and announced to everyone that Lolita's half-siblings had been removed from the natural mother's home for the same reason Lolita was. The natural mother was selling sexual favors from her young children in exchange for drug money and permission to stay in a house full of drug addicts. The authorities had been alerted by a family member who recognized disturbing phrases from the four-year-old.

Our concern for our deaf children is that if no one in the family can communicate with them, then how can they recognize the "disturbing phrases"?

Around 90% of deaf children are born to hearing parents.
Most of those parents never learn to sign.
It is not uncommon for deaf children of hearing parents
to come to school having no language skills at a time
when they are expected to learn content
like science and social studies.
Some children don't know their own names.

One day in a home ec. class, we watched a video on nutrition. The film was a brief documentary interviewing dancers and models. The video was to my back, so I couldn't see the images. After class, Lolita started pelvic thrusts while walking down the hallway. She said the people were naked and dancing like that. During the next class period, she peed on herself sitting in class. I later learned that was her orgasmic response.

The next day she played on the computer, a paper doll dress-up game.

Later that day she peed on herself.

The counselor came and determined that the dress-up game in underclothes was the catalyst for her to pee because that is her orgasm.

On occasion the lunch ladies told me that Lolita often "gets down" and "does pelvic thrusts" and "gyrates" in the lunch room while standing in line. They said that the previous week was really bad and they told her to stop.

The home ec. teacher was quite distraught over the video because the curriculum still had sexual responsibility, sexually-transmitted diseases, and baby care. Actually, the Deaf education teacher had put her in the class because that class took home the baby dolls that are programmed for real-life situations. The home ec. teacher disagreed that taking home the baby was a good idea. Lolita couldn't hear when the baby cried. When she got angry, she would react violently. That computer-programmed baby was an expensive temper tantrum. The point of the assignment was to teach the students how much attention and responsibility is associated with childcare and to dissuade sexual activity.

Lolita was incapable of understanding all of this. In fact, my greatest fear was quickly becoming that she would conceive. She did not understand that sex led to pregnancy, or that pregnancy was painful and uncomfortable, or that babies and baby dolls were not the same.

The deaf education teacher's decision prevailed and Lolita remained in the class. The home ec. teacher's decision was to not allow Lolita to take home a baby and send her out of the room on the frequent occasions when topics inappropriate for her were being discussed.

Chad

One day in the second week of school, Chad and I were on our way to class when he said he needed to go to the bathroom. He went in and I stood in the hallway by the door. Other boys went in and out, some gave me a significant stare. Chad didn't return. I leaned in the doorway. There he stood, with pants around his ankles, underwear around his knees, shoes under one arm and his bag under the other. He was walking out to find me. He was half naked. He couldn't sign because his bag was in his arms. I took the bag from him. He signed in a panic, "Dirty. Nothing. Don't want. No clothes." I signed that he needed to pull up his pants because he couldn't leave like that. He became very agitated, panicky, and said they were gross and dirty and didn't want them. I signed, "You stay. I find something. Stay here. No leave." I went to the office to get help with supplies. All they had were girl's shorts and no underwear. He became very angry because there was no clean underwear and he did not want to wear the dirty underwear.

Later when I reported the incident to the deaf education teacher and counselor, they laughed, gave each other a conspiratorial smile and said, "Well, at least he didn't do what he did last year! Last year he went streaking through the parking lot!"

I said, "He would have if I hadn't gone in to check on him!"

"That is nothing compared to what he did before…Just don't let him leave the bathroom."

Now an interpreter's job is to facilitate communication. That's all. Technically, an interpreter is not to give orders to a student ever. The deaf students have to be allowed to make decisions, just like any other hearing student, without fear of the person who is providing communication services.

Similar bathroom incidents occurred two more times before the end of the school year.

He went to the bathroom in the clinic. I stayed close by, but the room was also where students received their meds and checked blood sugar, so it was an active place. I heard a Deaf-yell from the bathroom. Chad opened the door and stood naked from the waist down. His wet pants lay on the floor. He said he needed his backpack. I advised that he get dressed to retrieve it. He dressed and I watched him leave the office and walk the wrong way down the hallway while I was relaying the situation to the nurse. When I went after Chad, he was on his way back to the office, wobbly, saying he was confused and didn't know where his locker was. We went together to get his backpack. He changed clothes while I looked for bags for his dirty clothes. He lay in the clinic and fell asleep.

Susie

Susie sat alone at a table in front of the room. By fifth period, she had met her focus and learning limit and could no longer sit still. She was ready for lunch.

The teacher talked about teen topics: anorexia, bulimia, teen pregnancy, and budgeting.

I interpreted.

Susie primped: lip gloss, fingernail polish, and ponytail up. Ponytail down. Ponytail up. Ponytail holder got stuck. She started to get upset. Panicked. Near hysteria. Since the interpreting was pointless, I encouraged her to ask the teacher for help.

As an interpreter, I can cause many extra problems if I break role. For me to take care of her, I establish myself as a caregiver and babysitter. Then the teacher wouldn't know what issues the student had. It is when the teacher/administrator/ counselor does not take care of issues that real problems arise.

Susie refused to ask the teacher. She looked for scissors and couldn't find them. She pulled the ponytail out with a wad of hair in it.

The following week Susie showed up at school with the front of her hair clipped to the roots. She said it bothered her so she cut it off. Then distressed, she said, "Mom said I am ugly. Boys not like me, not think me pretty. Me pretty? Boys not like me?"

Cal

Isolation is a defining characteristic of many deaf students who are mainstreamed. It is not isolation like solitude. It is solitary confinement. It causes many psychological issues in addition to the ones they may have from their home lives. One deaf educator told me that she has asked students through the years if they could magically become hearing would they. Most answer no, but of the ones who answer yes, most of them are boys. The boys seem to feel the isolation more keenly than the girls.

One day during a Guidance period, the school counselor discussed peer pressure and inclusion with the class. She emphasized that the students should be aware of others and notice if someone is sitting alone at lunch, to include new students and not ignore them. She asked for empathetic responses from the class. After all of the class had responded, Cal raised his hand and signed, "Me sit by myself at lunch. I am sad. I want friends. Then one time my friend Chloe sat with me. That made me happy. She is my best friend."

We left early for lunch because Cal took meds every day. The teacher said that when we left, the class discussed his comments. Some cried. All felt sad and guilty. She said it was a perfect teachable moment and she encouraged the class to include Cal and not let him sit alone at lunch.

The next two days Cal had company at his lunch table, but it didn't last. He said, "I eat and all of the people went like this" then he pushed back an imaginary chair from an imaginary table with a look of disgust on his face and plugged his ears. He continued, "Why they do that?"

I signed, "Maybe you eat with your mouth open. If they are plugging their ears, maybe it means you make loud noises when you chew."

"But why they do that?"

I said, "Do you remember last week when you were helping put chairs on the tables in the cafeteria and you touched the gum underneath the seats? Do you remember how you gagged and said, 'Gross!'? Same thing."

"Yes, but why they do this?" and repeated the acting performance.

Teachable moment over.

Amy

Amy was an intelligent young lady who was deaf and had experienced abuse. Like most deaf, her family did not sign. She became a behavior problem and acted inappropriately for a normal school setting.

Amy, however, was one of the few who were given an opportunity for rehabilitation in a facility that caters to the deaf – where the staff signs. It is called the National Deaf Academy in Florida. The facility is a school, a boarding house, and a counseling/rehabilitation center. It was a perfect solution…except it was expensive.

At one time, the states helped shoulder the cost, but when budget crises arise, policies change. The cost reverted to the specific counties. Rural counties cannot afford such a facility, so some students were sent back home for lack of funds.

Now many states have facilities for people who have various disabilities, physical or intellectual, but most states don't also have a staff who knows sign language. So communication frustrations manifest themselves in bad behaviors. And for a twenty-year-old, those bad behaviors can have violent results.

Amy aged out of the system at 22 years old. She went home. To an aging, and scared mother who had no idea how to handle her violent, frustrated daughter.

Since writing this, we have learned of the closing of the National Deaf Academy for allegations of abuse. The link is below of the news report by Aliza Nadi with NBC News.

http://www.nbcnews.com/news/us-news/national-deaf-academy-hit-abuse-allegations-closing-n497516

Al

Some deaf children, like any child, have the charming smile and demeanor of an Eddie Haskell. They look sweet, handsome, and vulnerable because of their disability. The truth behind the smile is that they are clever in deception and use their keen sense of vision and slight-of-hand to take things that do not belong to them. Sometimes it is just because it is a game to them. Other times it is because they really want to steal something for themselves.

Al was one of those kids. He stole a flash drive from science class. I don't think he actually knew how to use it, but he saw it and saw that he could get away with it. It wasn't a student's; it was the teacher's. And the teacher wanted it back. A major recon mission was deployed. No one in school was allowed to change classes until the perpetrator was caught. The principal and vice principal stood in the room and gave the lecture. Pockets were turned out. Book bags were emptied. I had a sneaking suspicion that it was the student to whom I was assigned because he had been asking about the object and stared at it quite a bit. I asked him if he had it. He said no with such a precious, innocent face which communicated to me that he was offended that I would suspect him, a perfect angel.

Sure enough. After an hour, it came out of his shirt sleeve.

He had hidden it and lied about it. He never showed remorse.

But what punishment was there? School rules require In-School-Suspension (ISS). He was isolated all day, every day. ISS was just a location change, not a punishment, and certainly not a teachable moment.

The reason the flash drive had been laying on the table to begin with was because the class had a technology presentation. Projects like this wouldn't normally stress me so much because a middle school student should be responsible enough to take ownership of his/her own work. All of the other middle school students were. Of course, Al wasn't normal. And like many students, Al didn't have a guardian to help with projects like that.

Al's technology project was a video phone which the Deaf can use to communicate by signing to each other. It is better than texting because English is such a struggle for many Deaf students. It would have been the perfect kind of project for a Deaf middle schooler except Al didn't have Deaf friends—or hearing friends for that matter—to whom he could communicate.

The idea for his presentation was for the workers at Tech Store to sign to Al in the classroom via the video phones. (I taught the employees sign to use with him.) That way Al had a nice presentation, but he was not really required to talk for the entire allotted time.

The big day arrived, Presentation Day. I had coordinated all times, plans, signs, and script with Tech Store employees, Al and the science teacher.

Then during 1st period announcements, they announced that there would be a pep rally at 9:30. Guess what time Tech Store was supposed to call? Yep. 9:30.

Al and I went to the science teacher after 1st period to ask about the presentation. She gave Al a new time. I left numerous messages with various people at Tech Store on Al's behalf, since there was not a video phone at the school. The science teacher had Al present during 4th period without Tech Store.

Horace

On the first day of school together, I took Horace a pencil with a Captain America eraser on it. As I interpreted a lecture on the Magna Carta, I watched him tear the eraser to pieces and eat it.

The next class was a math class where I learned that Horace could not count to 10. After that was a science class where the curriculum began with ionic and covalent bonds.

He didn't know what day it was. He took a modified quiz which asked what "religion" and "freedom of speech" meant. He didn't know so he copied the definition from the teacher's notes.

Normally his modified quizzes and tests were true/false or multiple-choice questions with only two choices. Horace would circle one of the two answers and turn it in. The teacher then graded it and gave the quiz back to him to correct. The answer was obviously the other, so he always had good grades having no idea whatsoever what any test or quiz was actually asking.

His social studies final for the previous year was 3 questions:
1. What city do you live in?
2. What state do you live in?
3. Do you live in China?

Those three questions required an entire year to get a correct answer. He apparently was determined that he lived in China.

Even the best of days were studies in dysfunction. I interpreted lectures on state geography and cash crops. The teacher would pass out a blank map of the state for students to write in significant geographical markers.

Horace excitedly looked to me and said, "I know this place! I live here!"

"Yes!" I sign-screamed. "Yes! You do!"

"Do you live there, too?" he asked.

Science was a class which was very active with labs. In theory, that was perfect for a deaf student. Except this deaf student was bizarrely afraid of insects, fire, bad smells and sharp instruments. During most lectures, the student played and talked about his girlfriend. I voiced it hoping that the teacher would instruct him to be on task, but the teacher merely ignored it.

A fire drill sounded, so the class proceeded to go outside. Standing a safe distance from the building with the group of students who were instructed to remain silent, I observed Horace become quite agitated staring at the pavement and pointing. I walked closer and found an army of ants. His bizarre reaction was something I had never witnessed, even with young children when they showed fear of insects. He didn't crush them, but he wouldn't walk away either. He walked around, hovering and very agitated. Fortunately, we were allowed back inside soon after. But we would revisit the insect issue again.

The class had a pet iguana which they fed live crickets. The crickets were kept in a separate cage. Live. Walking around.

During a lecture on endothermic and exothermic reaction, Horace was obsessed watching the crickets. He raised his hand. I always cringed when he commented in class because he could blurt out any crazy thing that I would be forced to voice. This time I thought that surely the teacher would do something to bring him back on track.

Horace: Why are the bugs there?

Teacher: We feed the iguana with them.

Horace: But they can crawl out!! Take them out and kill them!!

Teacher: Oh, they are harmless. See?

She proceeded to take the bugs to the center of the room where the class engaged in talk of bugs…far from the topic of the day—igniting matches and condensation.

All of this in itself is not anything over which to raise concern except for the fact that this child is nearing driving age and mainstreamed. This child and others like him were not in classes that taught him how to survive after school. This child was never going to college, yet he was in classes that were in theory preparing him for college. I have heard many defenders of this teaching philosophy say that it provides behavior models for the special needs children and provides the regular education students exposure to those with special needs. Each of those points is valid, yet I have dealt with the outcome of that philosophy to the point where we have deaf on the streets, homeless. Where is the value in that?

I have heard a school administrator say that deaf children are expensive children. I have also heard that some of the deaf students who age out of the school system land in state programs for behavior modification, counseling, job readiness training, and life skills classes costing the state half a million dollars a year. With all of that money invested in the deaf person, she should have super-human skills and wear a cape. …so what happened?

Who is responsible for the decision to put the student in such circumstances? Horace had seen countless different interpreters, deaf education teachers, and administrators in his short life. Each deaf education teacher had a different philosophy. Most, if not all, administrators had no knowledge of deaf children or education of deaf children. The deaf education teachers and interpreters were a constant revolving door. And why? Decisions were being made that had no knowledge or background to support them. Those hiring interpreters or teachers had no knowledge or experience to wisely hire either. Those who worked in deaf education were constantly micro-managed and lived with constant fear of being punished or fired, so they did jobs unbefitting their conscience and accepted unfair treatment.

The deaf I knew growing up were all literate, gainfully employed, for the most part happily married adults with families. Since then, I have seen major changes in deaf education, heard the research that supports it, yet I see the deaf children who cannot send an intelligible text or email. I see a disconnect, but I am not sure why. I was recently talking to a friend who works at a school for the deaf and she told me that she thinks it is the lack of language. Period. Our deaf children do not have a community of people around them who can communicate with them. They do not have access to language in any language at any level. I know that the trend has been to close the schools for the deaf, and the Deaf community has been outraged over it, but it is more than just because their childhood home is destroyed. Language is a lifeline. And in this case, a literacy line.

A friend of mine who is a certified interpreter came up with a plan to help the education of the deaf children and presented the plan to the school board of her county, proving how an administrator over the interpreters would be cost effective for the county. They agreed and created a position just for her. She has revolutionized deaf education in her area. Families with deaf children move to the county just so that their children can be under her care. More than that, she serves as a valuable resource for the teachers who work with Deaf students. When they have questions, they call her. When other counties have questions, they call her. She is an example of how someone at the administrative level, who is qualified and professional, can benefit the children and the school systems. Now there is still work to be done. Not all problems have been solved, but it is surely a good place to start.

Maybe mainstreaming is the best answer. Maybe a school for the Deaf is the best answer. With the national average reading scores less than 4th grade, maybe we don't have the answers yet. But finding what DOES work and building on that must be a priority in education.

Horace is a mainstreamed Deaf student in a hearing, public school.

An example of a day with Horace:

1st period – Horace took a modified quiz (like the one above) and made a 100%

2nd period – He was unable to add 13+1. He could draw 13 lines and 1 line, but was unable to make that 14.

He wrote "4 pennies+ 2 nickels= 2" and "3 pennies+ 2"

Horace couldn't distinguish between addition and subtraction problems.

3rd – The assignment was to balance chemical equations on the computer. He couldn't.

4th– While the teacher discussed checking accounts and investments with the class, Horace worked on worksheets identifying money and adding them.

5th – Interpreter administered the mid-term exam. Horace struggled identifying nouns and verbs.

He wore sunglasses through class. Soon to get his driver's license.

Charles

One week in history class, the teacher slides in a movie about the Incas and the Aztecs. Movies pose a special issue for interpreters because typically the lights are out so that the student can't see the interpreter, rarely do the interpreters get to see the movie ahead of time, and the movies are rarely closed-captioned. Of course, closed-captioning only helps those deaf who can read anyway.

In this case, there was enough light coming through the window that the students could see the interpreter as he was standing in front of the television. The picture was to the interpreter's back.

The Inca-Aztec war was rather gory. The interpreter couldn't see the pictures behind him, but the story was about two brothers, each on an enemy army. One defeated the other and the victor ate soup out of his dead brother's skull. The interpreter was unaware of the graphics that were on the screen, but the interpreter noted the reaction of every student in the room. They were all covering their faces, turning their heads, or wrinkling up the noses in disgust—

everyone but one. Charles sat facing the interpreter with absolute euphoria on his face.

In the next class he sat masturbating under his desk.

The interpreter later learned that Charles had a history of torturing animals. Cats had disappeared from his home frequently. The dog he currently owned had endured quite a bit of torture, all of which had been documented by children's services.

First periods, especially Mondays, were chocked-full of surprises. Since the interpreter was the only person in Charles's life who could communicate with him, he bottled up every shocking event and confusing emotion, shook it all up during the weekend separation, and let it explode when he caught sight of him. Very often that would be in a packed hallway of teenage students gathering their things for class. Charles's signs would be screaming down the hallway over the bustle of activity around. He would be in a panic and signing in hysteria, "Brother throw clothes!!" "Cousin stole ball!!" If the interpreter didn't meet up with him before the class began, the conversation would leak out during class time. The interpreter should have voiced all of it from the beginning. But he didn't. Ninety-nine percent of the time the teacher would not be near when Charles signed salacious stories, so the interpreter warred with whether or not he should voice them. Did he really need or want to voice what Charles was saying? The kids could do nothing but tease him or be scared of him. How could they ever be friends if they knew what occupied his thoughts all day every day? The interpreter chose to hold it until he saw the deaf education teacher. By the end of the year, he changed his decision.

One day Charles came to school and told the interpreter he had scooped up his pet turtle, flipped it onto the table and smashed it with his bare hands. Then he played doctor with it. Over and over and over he described the scene to the interpreter with more detail each time. That day in science class he was to dissect a frog. The interpreter had grave concerns, but according to school rules he was only allowed to tell the deaf education teacher what he had been told. When Charles and the interpreter arrived in class, he took the teacher aside, and as diplomatically as possible tried to impress upon her that he had concerns. She stopped the interpreter abruptly and told him to tell the principal. The student and the interpreter proceeded to the office. The nurse sat with the student while the interpreter went to see the principal. He asked the principal if she knew that this student had a history of animal torture. She said she did not. The interpreter explained to her the story of the student and the turtle.

She laughed.

She said that the interpreter was to go to the library with the student for the rest of the day. The interpreter asked if she would at least come into the library to check on the student. She said she would. She never did.

That day, for the rest of the day, the student was bored and continued to relive the animal killing. The interpreter told himself that he only had to make it to the last bell of the day. Just a few more hours.

There was a tornado that day. They had to go into the library's inner sanctuary for two hours after school. The school was on lockdown until the danger of the storm had passed.

The following day the deaf education teacher was back as well as the school counselor. The interpreter told them the story of the turtle as he was supposed to do according to school rules. Both of them laughed at the interpreter and said, "It really is funny. You have just been in regular education too long."

(The interpreter was not trained in any medical capacity or psychological capacity.)

The school counselor said that Charles had met his limit. Whatever his condition was, he would only get worse. His conscience was disappearing. He could no longer distinguish between right and wrong.

Not too long after that incident, Charles went to a party with another deaf friend. The following Monday, Charles came into school before first period and told the interpreter that he and his new deaf friend had sex, and that they had plotted to kill his friend's parents so that they could have sex all of the time.

This was so out of his pay grade.

The deaf education teacher was not on campus yet, and after the principal's overwhelming lack of support, he was not going there. So, he sent a 911 text to the deaf education teacher and counselor and when they arrived the student and interpreter were called to their room. A report was given and a three-hour counseling session began.

The next three hours were quite intense as the interpreter relayed some graphic sexual encounters as well as a detailed plot that the boys had hatched to kill the parents. It involved a hatchet.

The counselor alerted the proper authorities and the interpreter was told not to say or do anything. He was not to have any contact with Charles's family nor the other boy's family. But because he knew something of criminal law, he knew that action had to be taken in 24 hours. He did not expect Charles to be at school the next day.

Charles was at school the next day.

And the next.

And the next.

And the next.

He was told he could do nothing. When he asked about the reason, he was told that child services did not have an interpreter.

So he printed a list off and gave it to the counselor.

Child services said they had to be state approved.

He told them they were state approved.

Two weeks went by. A detective came to interview the student at school. No interpreter.

Another day went by.

He was told to interpret. He refused. He was told that the school attorneys had assured them that he would be protected and that he could interpret. He knew differently. He refused. The deaf education teacher interpreted.

The truth is that learning sign language is not a requirement to become a deaf education teacher. They are not required to learn it, much less become certified in ASL.

The decision was that no evidence could be found to prove what had occurred, so the result was that the two families were angry with each other for accusing the other and the boys never saw each other again.

When the interpreter saw that no effective changes were being made, he decided to do what he should have done from the beginning. He started voicing absolutely everything that the student signed.

Within one week, he was moved to another school. The student remained.

Jackie

Many special education classes have unique dynamics because its inhabitants are not in high school, yet in high school. The students are allowed to remain in special education classes until age 22.

That is also true in the alternative schools. Alternative schools here are the schools where students are sent if they have misbehaved so badly that they cannot stay in the general population, but their behavior is not so bad that they were placed in prison.

One of those students was deaf.

Her name was Jackie. Jackie, according to interpreters who had worked with her for years, was not a bad kid. She was typical of some deaf in that when she had trouble communicating, she became more aggressive in her behavior in order to express herself. But as long as she could communicate, she was sweeter than any student on the planet. She was also a foster child and over the age of 18; therefore, she fell under the oversight of the adult services program. Jackie was a favorite of those who worked in deaf ed. She was sweet, funny, very smart. She had just been dealt a lousy lot in life. She was the product of her country environment. She wore blue jeans, cowboy boots, and a big belt buckle every day. She trusted the people in deaf education. And they loved her.

One day she came to school and told the interpreter that drug deals had been going on at home. She had frequently alluded to such goings on, but this time she had specific days, times, and descriptions. Because she was in state custody, the school alerted the adult services.

The next day Jackie didn't come to school.

Nor the next day.

When the school inquired after her, they were told that adult services called the home to alert them that they would be coming in the next two weeks. When they did arrive, Jackie wasn't there. In fact, the foster family said that Jackie was visiting distant family and wouldn't be back for a while.

Jackie was never heard from again. Because she was over eighteen years old, there was nothing they could do.

The interpreter later learned that the family who had Jackie had no gainful employment. Jackie was the only money they had coming in...other than the alleged drug deals.

Harley

Little Harley looked like Buffy from the 70s TV show *Family Affair*. She had blonde curly hair in pigtails. She was always grinning and bubbly. She even had a doll like Mrs. Beasley.

Little Harley also had cochlear implants and a family that was loving and supportive. Harley's mom was a highly educated woman who worked for a local research hospital. The hospital had a new cochlear implant study and preschool program that Harley was eligible to be a part of. So Harley from her earliest years had exposure to language and extensive training in speech and sound. She had the best there was to offer in expert advice and resources. And she had a mom who drove her to school and doctor's appointments every day, a two-hour drive.

Once in elementary school, Harley's parents worked closely with the teachers and administration to make sure that Harley's needs were being met. And Harley was successful in school, both with academics and socially. Because Harley sometimes struggled hearing everything in the classroom, her parents worked with her every night on her homework and re-taught anything that she had struggled to hear in the classroom.

> Marc Marschark says in *Raising and Educating a Deaf Child* that
> …there has never been [any] real evidence that learning to sign
> interferes with deaf children's learning to speak.
> In fact, early sign language consistently has been shown
> to have beneficial effects on learning spoken language.
> Meanwhile, exposure only to spoken language typically results
> in significant delays in language development
> from early childhood continuing through high school years
> (Calderon & Greenberg, 1997; Geers, 2006). (Marschark 4)

The parents also wanted Harley to learn sign language for the eventuality when the technology was not working or when the cochlear implant was not on, like when she went to bed or went swimming. The school system refused to teach sign language to the oral child, so the parents paid for classes and tutors outside of the school system.

All of this set-up Harley for success as she entered middle school.

The only difference is that in middle school, there is not just one teacher with whom to make accommodations. There are seven teachers, and a group of students who are noisier and rowdier.

Harley found that in middle school, teachers would forget that they needed to face Harley when they were speaking. They would give entire lessons talking to the board while writing sentences, notes, or math problems. Power point presentations were made with the lights out and the teacher next to the computer to change slides while speaking from the back of the room.

With all of the energy required to listen intently, block out residual noise, and strain the eyes to read faces in the dark, Harley arrived home after a day at school absolutely exhausted and unable to stay awake long enough to be re-taught the day's lessons by mom and dad.

A Deaf Education teacher once told me that in her 30 years' experience, she found the children who were hard of hearing were at higher risk than those who were profoundly deaf, for a few reasons. One reason was because many students who are hard of hearing are not identified. They are actually labeled as discipline problems, rebellious, or disrespectful for not responding when given direct orders. She said that many students in In School Suspension (ISS) were actually students with hearing loss. Those students were at risk of dropping out of school.

Another reason that she said the hard of hearing children had a more difficult experience in school is because people assume that since they can hear some, read lips, and speak that they are hearing. They assume that the students do not need any other accommodations. They will turn their backs on the students, speak at a fast rate of speed, or yell at them from across the room. Many of these children when they grow up will simply identify themselves as Deaf because it makes life simpler.

One student was diagnosed in first grade as learning disabled based on scoring of tests and put in special education classes. The child endured all of the persecution through school that special education students often face, and he worked very hard to do well in school. When he was a senior, he went to the doctor for all of the medical exams required before going to college. The doctor performed a different hearing test than what had been done before and found out that the child was not disabled intellectually at all, but, in fact, had significant hearing loss. They fitted him for hearing aids and he heard for the first time in his life. On the way home while talking with mom, he started laughing and said, "I didn't know farts made a sound!"

At school the next day, he cried because he heard the National Anthem for the first time. He hadn't realized he wasn't hearing it.

Mary

Mary was a sweet, beautiful, innocent seventeen-year-old senior in an inner- city high school. She was in a school system where all of the Deaf in the county were bused to one school for services, so she was a long way from home. She wore modest, clean clothes which were in stark contrast to the students around her who were dressed much like Victoria Secret models. Mary always wore her hair in a ponytail and little if any make-up. She was always polite and gracious to students around her, teachers, and interpreters. Interpreters were thrilled to be assigned to interpret for her because she was so pleasant and kind.

During down time in class, I would start-up casual conversation with students, and this particular day I talked to Mary about her senior year and plans for the fast-approaching college days. She said that she was planning on going to a state school where there was a large Deaf group of students and many accommodations. Her plan was to major in early childhood development. She said that she was very much looking forward to the weekend because she was turning eighteen. I asked if she was the only deaf in the family, and if her parents knew sign, if a lot of people were coming to her house to celebrate the big day. She said she was the only deaf, her parents didn't sign and that her parents didn't usually have a big party, but she was eager for the coming big day because she could have sex.

She continued that she was not allowed to have sex because she was under eighteen, but now that she was having the big birthday, she could have sex. Then she was headed to college and she could have sex with lots of boys there.

Mercedes

Mercedes was a typical teenager in most respects. She loved

jewelry, nice clothes, cool cars, and boys. She loved school only because there were dances that she could attend where she could buy a fancy dress and hang out with everyone else from school who were also fancily dressed. A full conversation with her often revolved around shoes, bags, nail polish, hair accessories…where they were bought, what color options there were and how much they cost.

We went to the homecoming game her junior year because she was part of a club whose responsibility was to pass out programs at the gate. When time came for the homecoming festivities, we all lined up around the gate to watch.

The homecoming court all came out with the girls in their formal gowns: floor length, Cinderella skirts, and bejeweled. Mercedes was in awe. She asked so many questions. Who were these girls? Why were they out there? What were they doing? Why did they have on those dresses? Why were they all in one color except for that one? I said that the girl in white was the queen. She was about to be crowned by last year's queen.

Mercedes's questions came more furiously then. Why was there a queen? There was only supposed to be a prom queen. When had they started crowning queens at homecoming? Who was last year's queen? Where was she?

I was thinking to myself that Mercedes had been at this school for three years. She had been in class when the homecoming courts had been voted on. What in the world did she think she was doing in those classes? What did she think was going on at the pep rallies when the girls on the court were called out and introduced? Had she not wondered about any of the crazy activities revolving around homecoming? Had she not been part of the parades with the girls riding on cars? Had she never been to homecoming games before? I knew she had because I had been with her. Had she not seen the girls then? How much of her high school experience in this mainstream school had just blown right by her? How much of the Americana experience did this American teenager never know existed?

Annie

Annie is a sweet child. She probably once looked like the Gerber baby with big round bright eyes and chubby little cheeks. Her broken home and dysfunctional home life had dulled the spark and thinned the cheeks. She was still a child with child-like innocence. Her eyes would laugh through the ropes of stringy hair in her face.

She lived with family, though not mom and dad. She had never met her dad and been taken away from mom because mom was frequently in jail for stealing. Annie had a strained relationship with her mom because mom had stolen from her. Annie didn't like mom stealing from her, so she was leery of her when she came around. Instead she lived with Grandma who was aging and in ill health. Annie at her tender age of nine was an emotional and mental mess…and she was deaf.

November of that school year saw many stresses in Annie's life that negatively affected her school work. Her mom had been coming around as of late, and that led to the eventual stealing and police and uproar at home. Grandma decided that it was the perfect time to introduce Annie to her dad for the first time.

She showed up at school on Monday as happy as I had ever seen her. She was glowing. She had on a new ring that he had given her, a flower and a sea shell. She talked about her sister that he had brought with him for her to meet. Her dad had told her that he loved her, he was glad to finally meet her, and that they would spend every weekend and holiday together from then on.

She even took her gifts around school to show everyone in the office and cafeteria.

The next day she was sad because she missed her dad. She spent all day writing letters to him and her new sister.

The next day she cried because she missed her dad and sister.

The next day she said she was very sick and needed to go home. She was sent to the nurse to lie down in the clinic. While we are alone in the clinic, she told me that when she got home, her dad would come over and make her feel better.

The nurse had me call home to Grandma. Grandma said if she wasn't better in thirty minutes that she would come to get her. Annie fell asleep. I called Grandma back, and she said that Annie's dad is not coming that weekend, but I am not to tell Annie.

The following week was much the same. Only intensified because Annie had not seen her dad and was distraught. By Wednesday, we were back in the clinic and Annie was sobbing. I was on the telephone with Grandma who said for me to tell Annie to stop crying because she would see her dad on Friday. (I knew this was probably not true, but signed it anyway. I knew that Monday morning would be traumatic.)

He did not show up.

This continued through Christmas.

He did not show up at Christmas.

Annie's birthday was coming up. At school we made her cupcakes, gave her presents, and gave her a birthday girl button that she wore for a week. She told us about her birthday party that was coming up and that her dad was supposed to come.

He didn't. But mom did. Annie returned to school angry because her family had gotten drunk at her party and fell off of the porch.

The next week she brought in a newspaper with a picture of her dad and his girlfriend on the front page. They had been caught cooking meth in their trailer. The police arrested the girlfriend, but Annie's dad was evading the police. She said, "Go, Dad, go! Get away from the pigs!"

Annie's half-sister was taken into protective services.

Tony

Tony was about eight and skinny as a bean pole. He was quiet and aloof at school. He came from a poor family with many siblings so his clothes were often hand-me-downs.

I learned that Tony didn't eat breakfast. He qualified for the free breakfast, but he did not arrive at school early enough to eat it. The DCS counselor said that he told dad that he needed to eat before he left, but then Tony fought dad because he only wanted to eat chocolate. He actually kicked and threw things at him.

He was always very hungry and ate everything he could get his hands on, including all of the food that other kids didn't want from their lunches and snacks. At a deaf picnic I saw him eat two double cheeseburgers, two bags of chips, three pieces of cake, and then pack his pockets and backpack full of candy and more chips.

One day at school Tony said his stomach hurt. I asked if maybe it was because of the new medication from the doctor the day before. He shrugged his shoulders. I asked if he had an interpreter at the doctor. He said no. I asked what kind of medication he had been given. He said, "Pink." Then the nurse asked Tony to eat crackers and water because he had not eaten breakfast.

Hallie and Barkley

I had never seen a fight before. Not really. Not fists making contact with flesh kind of fights. Until I interpreted at an inner-city school.

This particular class had two deaf kids I was responsible to interpret for, Hallie and Barkley. We were in gym class. Two classes had been combined this particular day and gym class wasn't actually going on. The kids were just hanging out in the gym. I was reclining against a wall with Hallie sitting near me. Barkley was across the gym with a group of guys. I was looking at my phone when I noticed a commotion nearby. I thought two kids were just horse-playing. And then I looked up. I saw the fist hit the face. Actually heard that sound. Sickening, flesh-mucking, fat-warbling sound. Two girls. One grabbed the other by the hair and started pulling. They came closer to Hallie and me. I leaned down and waved towards her face to get her attention. I signed, 'Hey, them. Close. We get out!'

Then she did something I never would have done or guessed that she would have done. She jumped up and joined the fight.

I stood in shock for only a second for I needed to find Barkley. I spotted him just as he came running to jump in the middle of the fight, too.

Huh. What was my role in this situation? I wasn't about to interpret that. And it was not my job to split up the fight. In fact, no teachers were around. I scooted along the wall towards the door. Two coaches came out of the back office and got the group under control.

But it left me with a question. What is the interpreter's responsibility in that situation? I can't honestly interpret for a student who thinks I will rat them out. But I also can't incite a fight.

I found the lead interpreter later and asked.

Her advice was this, when a fight breaks out, leave the room. Tell the student, you can come with me or you can stay. But I am leaving. The teachers know that the interpreter cannot be a disciplinarian. They know that they shouldn't leave the room with the interpreter alone.

Rudy

Some deaf children are just kids who cannot hear. Other deaf children have a variety of things going on AND they are deaf. I have heard it described as being just vanilla ice cream or being a sundae.

Rudy was a sundae. I never knew Rudy's actual diagnosis. I understand that others with his diagnosis rarely lived to age 18. In the meantime, Rudy had to be educated and clothed, fed, and kept safe. Rudy was also born into a split dysfunctional family.

Everyone in the school knew the child because every day started with the temper tantrum on the sidewalk. Bags thrown. Hearing aids torn up and thrown across the parking lot. Or hallway. Or cafeteria. Shoes came off and were thrown. Jackets came off and were thrown. Kicking, hissing, gnashing of teeth.

The child was mainstreamed, yet was pulled out of class for daily class time with the speech therapist – who was on another floor. And the behavior specialist – who was on another floor. And the deaf education teacher – who was on another floor. And the occupational therapist – who was on another floor. The child wasn't actually in the mainstream class for more than an hour every day. And as the interpreter who was assigned to accompany her on every transition, I witnessed her having breakdowns during transitions. Transitions were a problem. Yet Rudy was expected to transition at least once an hour to a different floor. How was the child supposed to be on grade level work? I voiced my opinion daily. Nothing changed. For two years. Interpreters were not allowed in the IEP meetings because they were not considered part of the educational team.

A new deaf education teacher came in the next year and said, "Hey, the transitions seem to be a problem. Why don't we cut down on those? And I don't think the child is performing on grade level. Why don't we try an inclusion class for special education and see how that works?"

Instantly, behavior problems stopped. Within a week, Rudy smiled and laughed for the first time since I had known him.

Then one day as I stood outside waiting on Rudy to arrive, I talked with the principal. School was starting. Rudy was late. We saw mom pull up to the curb. She slowed down, but never stopped. Rudy's door opened and he came stumbling out of the car. The car door swung until mom rounded the curve and gravity closed it. I looked up at the principal who turned around and walked away.

I heard years later that Rudy and his mom moved to another county. Within a week of moving to the other county and school system, Rudy was taken from the home and placed in foster care.

100

Humbert

One of our chocolate sundae kids who had a fractured home, tested the resolve of many around him. Humbert gave the deaf education teacher a note that said he touched his little cousin in the privates. The deaf education teacher called the counselor in. We were in the deaf education room the rest of the day while the counselor asked Humbert details of the incident. Humbert told the counselor through the interpreter that he put crayons in the hole of the cousin's privates.

The counselor reported the incident to the proper authorities and within a week a team of experts consisting of children's protective services, child advocates, attorneys, and a psychiatrist were assembled to determine what had happened and how to proceed. They told me I would be interpreting.

I refused, for many reasons, but mainly because I was not qualified in that I was not certified, and certainly not court certified. This was a meeting where the notes could certainly end up at trial, and no one but a court certified interpreter should handle that. Also, I knew the child too well as the classroom interpreter. And for all of the above, it was against interpreter code of ethics.

They said that they had checked with the school attorneys and that I would be fine to go ahead and interpret.

I still refused because it was ethically wrong and because I knew that if this situation went sour, I would be the first one offered up as scapegoat. I also thought that they would fire me for my decision.

They did not fire me for refusing.

They didn't acquire an interpreter at all. They used the child's deaf education teacher.

Now it is not uncommon for a deaf education teacher to have a bachelor's degree in deaf education and never take a sign language class. Fluency in, or even knowledge of, sign language is not required for that degree.

Nothing came from the meeting. The decision was made that there was not sufficient evidence to prove it had really happened.

About a year and many phone calls later, I was on the phone with an attorney who I learned was the one in that meeting. When we realized we were speaking of the same student, he said this to me:

"First of all, police officers aren't perfect people. They make mistakes."

In my head I was thinking, *Duh! That is not the point.*

"Second, not all parents are deserving of being parents."

Again, in my head I screamed, *DUH! Have you been listening to me??*

"And, listen, I have been doing this long enough, and seen enough people use sign language to know if someone really knows sign languarge or not."

I bit my tongue to stop myself from saying, I have seen *Law and Order* enough to know a real attorney when I see one, too.

Needless to say, nothing ever came of it. And that was my last hope.

Olive

Olive cussed like a sailor. I tried to match her colorful expressions, her intensity, but I don't think I ever did them justice. No teacher ever reprimanded her, or corrected her. I don't know if it was because of the school climate or because they didn't care or because they thought I was actually the one doing all of the cussing. Whatever the reason, she cussed a lot, which meant I did, too.

One day in a class of no more than ten students, Olive was in a cussing war with a young man. The two of them actually came up out of their seats and chased each other around the room spewing profanities and directives about each other's mother. I was right there with her. For thirty minutes. The classroom teacher was sitting quietly in a corner with a book. I kept looking at her to give her the look of "DO SOMETHING!" She never did. After thirty minutes, I gave it up too.

Olive ended up grabbing her stuff and walking out of class, and school. I sat in my chair until the bell rang. I was guessing I was not expected to ditch school with the student I was assigned to.

Cho

Some students that interpreters are assigned to make the interpreter eager for the assignment to be over. If the student is mean, then the interpreter spews meanness. But sometimes the students are so precious you want to wrap them up and take them home. Cho is one of those.

She was Chinese. Her family was poor. Cho always smelled of spices and the other deaf kids made fun of her and avoided her.

Cho is an example of a growing concern in the interpreting world. Her family does not speak English. In IEP meetings, a Chinese interpreter was required for the parents. For Cho, an ASL interpreter is required. Cho was in ESL classes with hearing students from Korea, India, and Africa.

Cho was a hard worker. She worked in the family business after school and did her homework to the perfection degree – as much as she could. All of the crazy disadvantages of a deaf child worsen exponentially when that deaf child has no language at all upon entering school at an advanced age and her family's language is not that of the dominant culture. No language that she was learning would ever match that of her family. But she had dreams. She wanted to go to college. She wanted to have a nice house and provide for her family. I just hoped she would have that chance.

Bridgett

Bridgett wanted to be an actress. She buddied up to the school drama directors. They all knew her name and had little private jokes they shared. The theater teachers brought her t-shirts and the Broadway Playbills. She actually wore the shirts on occasion.

Bridgett started getting into trouble with some friends of friends. They were stalking her and becoming more aggressive. Her friends encouraged her to talk to her teacher friends, but she never would. She was embarrassed and ashamed.

I broke my role one day and let it slip near one of the theater teachers. He then started asking questions and was able to advise her and get her help. Of course, she figured out that I was the one to rat on her so my rapport with her was destroyed.

George

George was a very studious young Deaf boy. He was a rule-follower and lover of all things in their proper place and order. He was the epitome of a Boy Scout in a place where there were no Boy Scouts. George came from a family that loved each other and parents that were invested in the lives of their children. George was the youngest of four and the second boy. The oldest sibling was also a boy, ten years older.

George's father was a gentleman who loved the Bible and took it to heart that his number one responsibility was to teach his children Scripture. Every night at the dinner table, the family took turns reading Scripture aloud. Even George was required to read aloud and not allowed to mispronounce words or skip words just because he was Deaf.

George and his brother shared a bedroom. They had two twin beds that were separated by a nightstand. At night George's brother would slip into his bed and touch him in ways that made George feel very uncomfortable. He didn't like it and told him to stop. His brother laughed and made fun of him. He bullied him into keeping quiet.

That worked for a while.

Eventually this Boy Scout got up his courage to tell his mom. The solution was to get the brother his own room. He soon left for college.

The DVD from Connecticut, *Do? Tell!* is a movie about four children who have been abused or neglected. It is all in American Sign Language and it encourages children to tell someone. Even if someone who is told doesn't do anything, tell someone else. It is made beautifully to communicate to children what to do without being too scary.

Louis

As an interpreter you spend a lot of time in someone else's mind. And if an interpreter is assigned to the same student for a long period of time, an odd connection can form- for better or worse. And if those two people are the only ones who can communicate the same language within the whole school, then a world starts to develop within the school that no one else is aware of. An interpreter can forget that not everyone around can "hear" the conversations happening.

For example, Louis was in a science class that was discussing different chemicals and their properties. Some of those properties were smell, color, and texture. The assignment of the day was to identify different chemicals by their characteristics. Each student applied a squirt of unlabeled liquid into numbered bubbles in their trays. Then they took the trays back to their seats and proceeded to fill out a chart identifying the liquids.

This was the kind of assignment that Louis loved. Hands on. Using senses that he was skilled in. He was the best smeller and seer in all of the school. So he took his turn in line to fill each bubble in his tray and went to his seat eager to prove that he was capable.

1. Liquid Dial Soap: orange. Slick yet thick. Smelled mildly clean.

2. Germ-X: clear. Slick and thick, yet not as thick as the soap. Acrid smell.

3. Dandruff Shampoo: blue. Thick and slick. Smelled clean.

And on they went…30 of them. There were a couple that gave Louis some trouble. One was clear yet it was close to some others that were clear and the smells were mingling. He raised his hand to ask help of the teacher, but she continued to pass by him. I didn't want to believe that it was on purpose, but I couldn't help wondering.

But Louis had answered so many other questions in the assignment and he needed to finish before the bell, so he asked me. I always try to stay away from helping the students with their work, because they cannot grow up depending on interpreters to help. They must be independent and do the work on their own or learn to ask the teacher/authority figure. We try to help them learn self-sufficiency and self-advocacy. In this case, the teacher was not helping and he was running out of time. So when he said, I think #17 is mouth wash, and I knew it was bleach, I said, "Um, maybe look at the other possibilities and their characteristics. What other options are there?"

"No. It can't be anything else. I think that one is bleach."

"Ok, then, write that down."

"But, no, then what is #20? I think #20 is mouthwash. I will taste it to see."

"NO!" I signed. "Don't taste it! What if it is bleach?" (I knew it was.)

"It isn't bleach!" He said. "I know it is mouthwash! I can smell it! See?"

Then Louis grabbed the sides of the tray to turn it up and smell the contents of bubble #20.

Now that moment lasted an eternity in my head. During a moment of conversation like that, I don't hear any outside noise. The conversation between me and Louis was growing in tension. As I saw him grab the sides of that tray, I imagined the liquids, including the bleach, pouring down the front of his clothing. I dove across the science lab table to grab the tray before it tipped over, and, unknown to me at the time, yelled the word aloud, "NOOOOOOO!"

I instantly realized that the room filled with other science students had been relatively quiet. No one was aware of the battle between me and Louis. I broke the quiet with my violent dash across the table and loud yell. All faces were looking at me as I held the tray to the table and Louis's red, angry face was staring at me, unaware of the other students. The teacher turned to glare at me, then turned back to the student she was attending.

Once I righted myself, I looked at Louis and signed, "You can't tip up the tray to smell, or the chemicals will spill down your shirt." He nodded and leaned down with his nose almost touching the bleach. He curled his nose and nodded. Yeah, it was bleach.

Later that year, a similar incident happened in the office. It was a day when the weather was threatening to get bad and many families were picking their kids up early from school. Louis's family was one of them. He was called to the office for early dismissal, so he packed up his stuff quickly and we proceeded to the office. When we got there, the office was full of other parents waiting. Louis's mom came up to me and said, "Louis, did you get everything you need? Did you remember your glasses?" (Mom doesn't sign well, so she lets me interpret.)

Louis signed, "No, I forgot. Let me go get them."

I knew he had put them in his bag, so I signed, "I saw you put them in there. You have them in your bag."

"No, I don't."

"But you do. I saw you put them in. Just open your bag and look."

"I don't want to look! I didn't get them!"

During this gestural exchange, Louis's signs were at screaming level. No one knew this but me. In my head his "voice" was booming loudly, ricocheting off of my inner skull. I forget at these moments that no one else is experiencing that but me.

I pointed to his bag and said, "LOOK!"

Then all faces turned to me and I realized that the room was quiet and I must have just voiced that as I signed it.

Louis did look. His glasses were there.

Alice

Alice once told me her dream was to work at the jewelry counter at Walmart. That is great, but it made me sad to think that that was as high as the sky was for her.

Then one day I told her that we had been working really hard to raise enough money to bring Lou Ferrigno to town to talk to us about growing up deaf and his experience with abuse. She had no idea who Lou Ferrigno was.

I said, "You know the big guy, green, in movies?"

"Yeah! Yeah! Yeah!" she signed.

"He is deaf like you. He used body building as his way to work through his anger and frustration and ended up in the movies."

In the next few minutes I could see her mind working. She then looked up at me and signed, "You know, I could work in the movies. I could maybe do hair and make-up for people in Hollywood."

"Yes!" I said. "Yes, you can do whatever you put your mind to!"

Johnna

One night I received a call from a local police department. A deaf young woman had run away from home. I knew the young lady, so I jumped in my car to see what I could do as an advocate for the deaf person.

When I arrived, the room was full of detectives and police officers scratching their heads. They were so relieved when I walked in. The deaf person was seated in a rolling chair, quite comfortable. The police officer was updating me on what was happening as she handed me the sheet of paper they had been using to write back and forth. I knew that this young lady had about a first grade reading level and even that was not in English word order. The words on the page were useless.

Since I was there as an advocate, the officer started asking questions to determine why the young lady was there and where she belonged.

The stories of mistreatment by family members through the years began to spill out.

The officer's mouth dropped.

She said, "I have never heard any of this before. I have been to the house many times for disturbances, but I never knew that the deaf child was a victim in all of this."

"Exactly." I said. "You have got to take an interpreter. You cannot let the family 'interpret'."

Well, no crime had been committed that night so there was nothing anyone could do. The young lady was 18, so child protective services could not be called. The family refused to take the young lady. There was no place for her to go.

I got in touch with a church in town that I knew often put people up for the night. They agreed to pay for one night. At least that would buy us some time.

I took the young lady to the hotel. They found out she was deaf and refused to let her stay. They said that if there was a fire they would be liable.

Normally in a case like that, I have a discussion with them about ADA and how it is their responsibility to supply accommodations with visual fire alarms and it is a violation of her rights to deny her. In this instance, I did not have the luxury of the conversation. It was close to midnight and we still had to shop for food and stuff for the night. I went down the road and paid double for a room.

Four months later, a similar incident occurred. This time when I called the church, they told me not to take them to that first hotel. I said to them, "You know that is against the law, right? They can't deny the deaf because they are deaf."

"Oh, honey, don't get so worked up about it. It isn't like they are denying him because of the color of his skin or something."

Yes, that is exactly what it is like.

After that particular night's events were over, I started an inquiry about how to handle it. I was advised to call the local disability law center. I had called them many times before on certain issues and was always told that I could not pursue the matter because I was not deaf and I was not a parent of the deaf child. The deaf would have to call themselves. In this particular case, the deaf person wasn't going to call because she had bigger issues to face.

I called the fire department and asked how they handled such situations. They said that they didn't. It is not the fire department's responsibility to make sure facilities are ADA compliant. What they did do was give me a visual alarm clock that doubled as a visual fire alarm that a hotel could use for deaf patrons.

I contacted a gentleman that I knew in the hotel industry and asked him how their company handled deaf patrons. He said that most hotel chains had an ADA box that they supplied for deaf customers so that the patron could use any room in the hotel and renting the room could be accommodated relatively easily.

The fire department and the law center both said that they would help me educate that hotel, and any others, so that they could become compliant. Making friends sounded much better than throwing law suits.

That particular night with the hotel also started a year-long battle to find a home for this young lady. I learned of a gaping hole in our system. There is no place for the deaf. Every place we called said that they could not take this person because she was deaf.

Vinny

A couple of our kids have ended up in jail. Whether or not they were really guilty of any crime is debatable since in every instance they did not have an interpreter.

I was in court with a friend who is a foster parent. She was in court to deal with her foster child. While I was there, I saw one of the deaf students I knew from school. He saw me and signed to me from across the room, "Can you help me? Can you interpret?"

I said," No, I cannot interpret in court, but I will see what I can do."

I walked over to Mom and said, "Hi. Vinny here asked if I could interpret today. Do you know if the court has an interpreter coming?"

The mom said, "Oh, yeah, I called for one and they should be here any minute."

I knew it wasn't true.

Sure enough, when the case was called, there was no interpreter. It is actually the court's responsibility, but it must be the parents who enforce it. In this case, the child was being charged with disturbance in the home. We interpreters knew that the disturbance was the parents, not the child. The parents didn't want his voice telling the truth in court. And it never did. Vinny left that day with a charge on his record.

Because this happens so frequently, the deaf often grow-up distrustful of the police. The police or first-responders may come to the home during domestic disturbances, but then take the deaf child to jail instead of the parents.

One such instance was with a young woman who found herself homeless. She had been kicked out of the family home and had nowhere to go. She had skills to support herself, but without a permanent residence, she couldn't get a job. She was taken by authorities to the local homeless shelter, but without an interpreter to explain the rules, she didn't know she was breaking rules. She was kicked out. It was fourteen degrees outside. She was cold and had no where to go. So she went to the closest, warmest place she could— the Ritz. Obviously, the Ritz wouldn't let her stay, but she had no where else to go. They called me and told me to come and get her. I was hours away and had no place to take her. I asked what they normally did with people like that. They said they called the police. I said that was what they had to do. So they did. The police arrived and called me. They told me I had to come get her. I told them I had no place to take her. Mobile Crisis couldn't take her because she wasn't suicidal. No other place would take her because she was deaf.

The officer ended up taking her to jail for trespassing. At least she was warm and fed.

The following day I found out what courtroom she was in and sat in the courtroom until her name came up on the docket. I found the public defender and intended to ask him to help us get her in front of the judge, hoping the judge could claim her mentally incapable of making decisions so that we could get her help. The public defender replied, "Oh, honey, don't worry about it. She plead guilty. She is going home today."

I closed my eyes and thought, 'Where do I start?'

I said, "So, you had an interpreter with you when she plead guilty?"

"Oh, no, we didn't need to call one. One of our security officers downstairs, his parents are deaf. Yeah, he helped us out with that. She is going home today."

I closed my eyes and prayed for wisdom and the right words to come out of my mouth. "She has no home to go to. I was hoping we could get her in front of a judge who could help us get her help."

The public defender looked at me and said, "Are you here to take her home?"

"No. She has no home."

"Are you here to interpret?"

"No, I am here as a friend."

"Then what good are you?"

I said, "She has no home to go to. She doesn't know what she is pleading to."

He said, "We are not a Holiday Inn. Her crime isn't even a crime. We can't fill up our cells with her. She is out of here today."

She was led into the courtroom with her hands in shackles. She tried to sign to me but struggled. She had to wait quite a while until the court interpreter arrived so that she could plead in front of the judge. When she walked to the stand, she asked the judge if she plead guilty if she was going home. The judge said, "Yes, Ma'am." So, she plead guilty.

I called her case worker when I left and told her what had transpired. She was livid. She said I was to call the law advocacy group for people with disabilities and tell them that her rights had been violated.

I told her that I had done that quite a few times already but what I had learned is that because I am not deaf, because I am not a parent of a deaf child, I can do nothing.

I called anyway.

They said, "The deaf person has to be the one to make the formal complaint. Encourage that person to make a formal complaint."

That was the whole point. She was unable to do so. She was homeless, first of all, and secondly, mentally unable to make such a motion.

A few weeks later, I had another phone call, this time from the emergency room. She had made it back home and another fight had erupted.

…Another night in a hotel. …Another morning with no place to go. One of the ladies at the hotel said to me, "What should we do with her?"

HOLY SMOKES!!! I had no place to take her.

I said, "You know, it is a beautiful day. Maybe she can go to the park or maybe sit by the lake."

She said, "She is not a dog."

I never said she was. But I had no place to take her. And I wasn't sure why in the world I was in trouble for her homeless condition. Why was her family not in trouble? Why, when they had the opportunity, didn't the school system help her? Why was I all of a sudden the bad guy?

We did get her to a safe place…for a while. In a few weeks, even that turned toxic. The lady who had her called me and said, "I have had it. She goes, or I do."

I was at my wit's end. I called my last hope. A state representative had been helping us with her case. I called him and said, "This awful situation is about to get so much worse."

He said, "Give me a few minutes and I will call you back."

He did.

He said, "I think I am learning what you have known for a long time. There is no place for the deaf in our state. No one will take her because she is deaf."

Three months later, with some string pulling, she found a home. The problem is, there are dozens more just like her.

The good thing is that a state representative had seen the problem first hand. Maybe help would come.

Marilyn

One night I received a call from a family with a deaf teenager. The young girl was refusing to eat, get out of bad, or do anything other than lie in bed and cry. Since the family didn't sign, they wanted me to come over and talk to her.

I have had suicide training for many years. Training on how to identify warning signs and then training in who to tell to get help. In this case, who makes house calls and speaks in ASL? I called some counselors I knew and threw myself at their mercy. I needed help. They gave me warning signs and trigger words…would that be the same for a deaf person? I didn't know. The answer was the emergency room if it was serious, or make an appointment with a counselor if it could wait. Did the family have insurance to cover it? I had no idea. I was really scared.

When I got to the house, I walked inside to find the child in question bathed, dressed, and sitting sweetly on the couch smiling at me.

The sad truth is that because of the isolation and lack of

communication with family members that many of the children face, mental health issues are a big problem in the Deaf world. And the number of mental health professionals who can help this group of people are so small that the Deaf do not have access to them.

There are a few groups who are addressing this need, like in Rochester, New York; however, I have found that it may as well be Egypt because the effect of the research and training takes too long to reach rural America. Too many of our Deaf are suffering from episodes just like Marilyn's that may not end so sweetly. We need more research and more professionals being trained and more people in the field effecting that change at a faster rate of speed.

Becky

A child in the rural South can expect dirt roads, blackberries, an occasional snake and the smell of honeysuckle. Summers are sticky, winters are mild. Tornadoes are a threat in fall and spring. Crossroads occasionally have a local farmer's fruit stand with tomatoes, corn, and peaches. These simple pleasures dot the memories even of those children who experience the most horrid of childhoods.

Becky grew up as one of those blackberry-eating children. She loved her momma, and her momma loved her. Becky was deaf in one ear and had a hearing aid in the other. Her momma worked with her every day teaching her how to speak and read lips. Neither Becky nor her mom signed because signing was discouraged, especially for children who were learning to speak. Becky's dad had left the family when Becky was a baby, and her momma re-married a man who worked infrequently and had an extended, close-knit family. Becky's momma was the main bread-winner in the family. The men of the house took care of Becky while her momma worked.

The men in Becky's household were her step-dad and step-grandfather. Her step-uncle and step-cousin lived next door. They shared a driveway and a woodshed. Her communication with the men was limited because she was deaf and just learning how to speak, but at age eight she understood when she was being told to do something she didn't want to do. And she understood fear from threats.

Step-dad had the easiest access to Becky because they lived in the same house. He could easily slip into her room after her mom left for work. He could force himself on her and threaten her with hurting her momma if she ratted him out. Then grandfather took interest and found that he could force her to the back of the woodshed after school for a quickie, also threatening to kill her momma if she told. Step-uncle and step-cousin were less aggressive in their abuse. They needn't threaten her with violence since the other two had her in hand. So they forced her to watch porn with them and provide services for their pleasure.

This was Becky's daily life from age 8 to age 16. Then one day Becky's mom noticed a stray hand on Becky, and Becky's grimaced expression. The next day Becky's mom intentionally came home from work early and found step-dad with her. That day Becky's mom took her away and divorced her husband.

Becky never dated. She did not feel comfortable around boys. Until the one she married. He didn't force himself on her, so she thought he was a good guy. After all, the only men she had ever known had forced themselves on her. Becky and her husband had two children together.

Once married, he started having affairs with other women. She accepted it as part of her life. He loved her and stayed with her, so she accepted his unfaithfulness. Then he met another, younger, Deaf girl and wanted to live with her instead.

Becky was crushed. She wanted to be loved for who she was.

She met other Deaf people and learned how to sign. She found that she felt comfortable with the Deaf. She also found that she felt comfortable with women. They didn't abuse her. They didn't force themselves on her. They loved her for who she was.

Layla

Layla was a beautiful young Deaf girl who was skilled at everything she put her hand to. She could swim, cook, sew and make friends with anyone. She even caught the eye of her teachers.

One teacher, a man, had taken a special interest in Layla. He invited her one spring afternoon to look at some flowers on the back side of a building near the playground. He took her hand and guided her to just the right spot. He told her how beautiful she was and offered to make her feel special. She shook her head no in protest, but he insisted and used his size to hold her still. He threatened her if she told.

Layla's grades which were once As and Bs became Ds and Fs. She did not want to go to school. She was frequently sick. A few weeks later the teacher again caught her outside and forced her around a corner. This time he had her skirt up, on the ground, when some boys heard her cries and came to investigate. The teacher heard them coming and left.

Summer came and Layla was free to be a child again.

The next year she heard he had gone to another school.

A few years later, Layla was in high school. She heard that they had a new administrator coming. It was the old teacher back again. This time he had an office. He called her to the office one day at the end of the school day. She did not want to go, but she could not disobey a principal. She went. And he made advances on her. This time she was bigger. She said no. She fought him. She got away.

Later that year he was caught making advances on another girl in the school just as he had Layla. He was moved to another school. Charges were never filed.

Laney

Laney was a bright, promising young child with curious eyes and an infectious smile. She liked to jump in puddles and make mud pies. She was like 25% of the Deaf children in the state; she went to the School for the Deaf. She left on Sunday afternoon and came home on Friday evening from the time she was four years old.

Laney loved her school. Everyone around her signed. Every teacher, every cafeteria worker, every administrator, every secretary, every garbage man...everyone could speak her language. She had so many friends who could sign that she couldn't even count them all. She went to football games and school plays, everything was in sign language. She was excelling in Reading, writing, math and science. She loved to learn and found no limits to her learning.

Then she went home.

Dad and mom didn't sign. But Dad did like to play games. He liked to play camp out and build tents in her room. He liked to play games and make her touch him, forcing her hand when she didn't want to play anymore. The games became more aggressive. The threats of harm to mother became more aggressive, too.

This pattern continued through every weekend, holiday, and summer vacation. One time at school, Laney went to talk to the school counselor because she desperately did not want to go home. Laney told the counselor about the "games" that Dad liked to play that she did not. The counselor alerted the authorities and an investigation began.

Eventually, the case ended up in court. No interpreters were provided. The judge found the father not guilty of any crime because there were no witnesses to confirm the allegation. Laney's mother was too afraid to leave her husband. Laney's life resumed the normal routine of school during the week and home on weekends, campouts and all.

As Laney got older, she started going to friends' houses on weekends and holidays. After she became 16-years-old, she could drive herself where ever she wanted to get away. Once she graduated, she never went home again.

Laney got a degree and a full-time job. Her skills and work ethic made her a valuable employee. However, her personal life was not so happy. She did not like the company of men, but she did want a baby. So she found a donor and had a baby.

Her baby girl grew up to be a smart, resourceful woman like her mom. She went to college to become a nurse. Laney's daughter never met her grandparents. The daughter was upset with Laney about not knowing her dad until she grew-up enough to understand her mother's experiences and reasons.

Sheila

Sheila is a chocolate sundae friend. How many of her chocolate sundae characteristics came from birth and how many came from abuse, no one will ever know. She is a lovely person. To see her no one would ever the guess the horrors that live so close to the surface. She was a beautiful baby girl with blonde, ringlet hair and round green eyes. She loved chocolate pudding with whipped cream and sprinkles more than anything in the world.

Sheila's parents divorced and Sheila was sent to her father's family to live. They resented having to take care of a deaf, disabled person. When they became angry, they swung bats at her to teach her a lesson. They stripped her naked and left her out in the cold for up to four days.

Sheila's mother eventually got word of what treatment she was receiving and went to get her. She found out that Sheila was pregnant. With her father's baby.

When the baby was born, Sheila's mother had the baby given up for adoption.

Sheila now suffers from PTSD. Most of the time Sheila is very happy, bubbly and smiling. She talks about the lovely weather, the pretty flowers, the frolicking hummingbirds, the tasty cake, but one trigger from her past and she is suddenly yelling and flailing. She weeps uncontrollably.

During all of the trauma years, no interpreters were ever provided. No charges were ever filed.

I had learned years ago what a shortage of interpreters there

Seventeen

Leap the Fence on Faith

"A song is rising from this place/With the world suspended in a state of nervous grace/But the harmony will give us what it's so hard to say/Out loud." (lines 25-28)

-Michael Higgins, "In This House"

was in rural areas and schools. I heard the side of the school systems and counties that said they didn't have the money to pay for the kind of interpreters that RID said were necessary. RID said that the best of interpreters should be in schools as language models, but few highly qualified interpreters are going to change dirty diapers and wipe snotty noses at barely over minimum wage. RID also has no authority to enforce their recommendations. Parents have that authority, but many of those parents have no idea what their rights are or how to go about enforcing them. Schools are facing budget crises and increasing demands with limited resources. Government agencies and law enforcement agencies face a myriad of demands with shrinking budgets and angry constituents. Each side stands in her corner of self-righteous indignation on her soap box spouting injustices while a world of Deaf children sit silently in classrooms. Those injustices of Deaf children become more severe when they leave American soil. Deaf children in many other countries face much worse than confusion in classrooms. Until we well-meaning adults can swallow our pride and be open to discussion, our children will continue to suffer.

I felt powerless to help these children. I witnessed or heard stories of these children and knew that as an interpreter I could not help. The phone calls and emails I sent were never returned. Doors were closed in my face.

I knew the moment I sat in my car overlooking the park at First Avenue, having hung up the phone with an attorney—my last chance at hope—that something had to change. Something. I had been searching for the person with answers and solutions, the leaders, organizations fighting for the kids. I couldn't find them. I was at that crossroads that we all eventually face at some point in our lives. It was that moment when you see the ruby slippers on your own feet and realize that the answer to the problem resides only within yourself. The moment when you look in the mirror and realize that YOU are the one who must make the change. ...I was scared. Scared isn't even the right word. It was a sickening feeling in the pit of my stomach, but at the same time a kind of resolve formed there, too. I didn't know how or where or what was next but I knew, as certain as the air I was breathing, that something had to change. Something that wasn't happening before. Something to make people not just hear words, but listen. I have since wondered if Harriet Beecher Stowe had a similar experience. Or the guy from. Or Ghandi.

Or Martin Luther. Or Martin Luther King, Jr. That moment when the cries, and screams, and pleas for help can no longer be ignored. When the thought of turning your life upside down and turning your back on all that is normal, comfortable, accepted, and routine feels like the preferable choice over living one more minute filling the cookie-cutter mold of what is accepted and status quo. Knowing that if I didn't do something then everything I had ever done or said in my life was a lie. I wouldn't be able to look at my children in the eyes and ask them to do anything again. This was my moment of decision. What did I really believe, and was I willing to give up everything for that belief?

Deaf history tells of a utopia for the deaf on Martha's Vineyard
in the 1700's. The island had an unusually large percentage
of deaf on the island, and everyone on the island signed
– both hearing and deaf. There was no distinction.
Deafness was simply a characteristic like
blonde hair or brown eyes or left-handed.
Deafness wasn't disabling.
It doesn't have to be now.

When I taught English classes, one of the pieces we studied was Martin Luther King Jr.'s "Letters from the Birmingham Jail". I have thought of lines from those letters often, when he said the days of "horse and buggy pace" are over (3). No longer will we wait. At that moment sitting in my car, I knew I could no longer wait. The time for running away was over. I had to accept what I needed to do.

And I knew the crazy girl that jumped the fence to get the ball was about to jump an even higher fence with much meaner Dobermans. But the fence had to be cleared. Had to be.

I took stock of what I knew and what I COULD do.

I could teach. I could teach children, college kids and adults. I could teach them sign language and Deaf culture. I had seen how effective it was when used in the classroom around Deaf children. I knew how successful the Deaf children could become when allowed to do so. I knew of resources in the Deaf world that rural areas were unable to access. I COULD do that. And if nothing else, those children would grow and become the decision makers to make the difference.

Some good things I knew…

1. Hands & Voices is a national organization made of parents of Deaf children. They work very hard to not choose a side of oral deaf or signing deaf. They want what is best for the child and the family. The National Hands & Voices has a program called O.U.R. Children's Project that helps parents whose children have been abused or who they fear could become a victim. Also, Hands & Voices works on a Deaf Child Bill of Rights (DCBR) in many states. This is what drew me to them. One of the pillars of the DCBR states that the deaf children will have people around them who can communicate in their language: peers, teachers, and staff. It also states that the deaf children have a right to deaf adults and mentors. (I am now a board advisor for the Tennessee chapter of Hands & Voices.)

2. Early Hearing Detection and Intervention (EHDI) recently helped pass a law requiring newborn screenings for hearing loss. This will help identify children sooner to help them get resources sooner.

3. Children of every age and gender love sign language. It is fascinating to them that their handshapes communicate. Like a secret code. And they aren't afraid to use it. For adults sign language looks like poetry in motion. They get choked-up and teary-eyed watching someone sign songs.

4. Most of the time, when people hear the statistics and situations that some deaf children face, they are outraged and want to know why something isn't being done.

5. Education is the key.

6. Language is a lifeline. We teach our kids to swim to keep them from drowning. We give them immunizations to avoid chicken pox. We can teach them language to avoid ignorance and isolation.

> Throw out the Lifeline across the dark wave;
> There is a brother whom
> Someone should save; Somebody's brother!
> O who then will dare To
> Throw out the Lifeline, His Peril to share?
> Throw out the Lifeline with hand quick and strong;
> Why do you tarry, why linger so long?

See!
He is sinking;
O hasten today- And Out with the lifeboat!
Away then away! (verses 1-2)
Edward S. Ufford, 1886, "Throw Out the Lifeline"

A friend who knew of my concerns through recent years advised me to stop running from the Deaf world. This is where I was supposed to be. This is where I was needed and where I had been planted for this reason. She had experience in the nonprofit world, so she walked me through the IRS 501 (c)3 paperwork, and the Sign Club Co. was born.

The dream for the Sign Club Co. was to re-create the Deaf Utopia of Martha's Vineyard from the late 1700's. A place where everyone could communicate in the same language. A place where a deaf person could walk into a store or post office and conduct normal business as easily as any hearing person with little or no inconvenience for anyone.

My focus was the children. I wanted to create an environment around the children like I had seen successful in that classroom where the teacher allowed me to teach sign language to the whole class. By the end of the year, I was rarely called upon to interpret for anything except direct classroom instruction. The child became a normal child. I wanted that for every deaf child.

If I could create little pockets of signing children in schools, then as a group, we could start teaching restaurants where we met for Silent Dinners. Then we could go to local entertainment venues like bowling alleys and arcades. I could make friends with the police department and local hospitals so that we could get basic information about Deaf culture to them, especially concerning our friends who were abused.

…that was the plan in 2012.

Then life took on hurricane status speeds.

The first school year we kept a few sign clubs we already had in schools and added a couple more. We had 5 clubs with about 150 kids. I taught all of them once a week either before or after school. We planned Silent Dinners every month at a different restaurant in town where we invited all of our Deaf friends and all of our sign language students to practice their new language with the people who owned it. We also planned a Deaf Abuse Awareness Day during abuse awareness month. The students in the sign clubs had a day of silence (approved by the teachers and principals). They wore their Sign Club shirts and a sticker with an abuse statistic on it. The kids made posters which were hung in the hallways. We all met at one of the schools on a Friday afternoon. A lady came to speak who was a victim of sexual abuse. The community relations police officer came and signed his opening remarks which I had recently taught him. He brought with him the K-9 and the bicycle cops. The Deaf were so excited to see a police officer signing: A police officer who said in their language, "I am your friend. Come to me if you are being hurt."

The next year we had eleven clubs. We filmed a few PSAs and brief sign language lessons which the local public access channel aired every Monday night. We decided to make a louder statement about the abuse, so we contacted the Guinness World Record organization about breaking a record. They suggested paper dolls. At that time the record was one-mile long. We thought, sure, 1 ½ miles is not so bad.

During that year, the record was broken twice so that by the time the next Deaf Abuse Awareness Day rolled around the record was four miles.

We did break the record that year on August 2 – our second attempt (wind is not a friend to paper dolls). We are now official Guinness World Record holders and have received a little more media coverage.

The five miles of paper dolls we then turned into two pieces of art to go on tour. One is a 4X6 frame of the famous paper dolls that includes a poem by Diane Brandehoof about abuse and the silence that a deaf child endures when she does not have an interpreter…like a paper doll.

The other artwork is a bridge made by Alan Danielson who has worked on movie sets. The bridge is able to be assembled and reassembled, walked around and under. It is covered with almost ten miles of paper dolls.

Those two pieces of artwork have continued the conversation about deaf children and abuse.

The third school year brought 16 sign clubs. I could no longer teach them all by myself and the advocacy was taking over. Of course, we had no money coming in. No granting agency would fund a nonprofit as young as ours with as little business experience as I had. Businesses in town didn't see a need to fund a program that dealt with deaf people.

The workload was increasing tenfold, however. The community

relations police officer who spoke at our first Deaf Abuse Awareness Day was also the man in charge of training for the town's officers. He set-up training in sign language and deaf culture for all officers in town. Then he introduced me to other chiefs in the county. One of those chiefs invited me to speak at the Association of Chief of Police meeting.

I was allowed ten minutes. I presented the need and asked for an opportunity to train all officers at in-services about the meager statistics of deaf children who are abused and the need for interpreters.

Before leaving that meeting, the Assistant Commissioner for the Department of Safety and Homeland Security came to me and said that he was interested in talking to me about making DVDs to train law enforcement across the state.

I received a phone call from one of the state senators who I had turned to for help. He was presenting a bill in the next legislative session about deaf children who are abused. He asked me to testify in front of state congressional committees.

On June 10, 2015, I witnessed the governor of Tennessee sign into law, the first of its kind in the nation, a law concerning deaf children who are abused.

A lady from Texas heard about the Sign Clubs and asked how she could have one at her school, too. Counties around Tennessee were calling asking the same thing.

The need is evident. The solution is simple: Language is a lifeline.

At every place I am asked to speak and tell our story, I find that the greatest support comes from interpreters. They **KNOW** that I speak truth. They have seen what I have seen and felt the same helplessness I have felt. They come to me with tear stains on their faces. They give me their business cards and offer their support whenever I need it. They thank me for speaking out about our deaf children and the struggles they face.

And it is not uncommon for me to receive phone calls from interpreters in the field who find themselves in a pickle and they are too afraid to blow the whistle so they ask for my help. That is why these stories are in these pages. The children's voices must be heard.

To date, the Sign Clubs have taught about 1500 people Deaf culture and sign language. Our mission is for everyone in our county to know one sign and every ballgame accommodated with the National

Anthem. Our vision is for every child to have a voice in school, with police and first-responders, and in court. Our goal is for every child to have a friend and role model. But more research is needed. More brilliant, creative, problem-solvers are needed to create solutions.

I once met a preacher from Northern Ireland who was known as the peace-maker in public meetings. He was frequently called upon to work his magic when turmoil started to bubble. He said to me, "Until we people of faith stop arguing amongst ourselves, we have no hope of reaching the lost world." I think that principle applies to many issues in our world. This sage of a man started building community groups where each member could share in the meetings a song, a cake, a poem, a sweater. Each learned to appreciate the other for his/ her talents and skills and stopped judging based on a pre-conceived stereotype.

…it is a beginning.

I don't know where this story ends, but I do know this: Last week at our Sign Camp, I had a deaf teenager sitting on my left when a hearing child walked up to my right. The deaf teenager signed to the child, "Have you had fun this week?" and the child signed back, "Yes, I had fun!"

A friend was made. A friend who is there for the laughs and for the tears. A friend who knows that the deaf are perceived to be a perfect victim if they do not have someone with whom they can communicate. A friend was made - through a shared language. We have hope for tomorrow.

> In this house, there are many doors
> And mine has a keyhole just like yours
> All the music needs is a place to begin
> In this house that we're all living in. (lines 29-32)
> -Michael Higgins, "In This House"

Love all! Keep signing!

Resources

My Favorite Resources

1. Hotline 1-800-222-4453. A toll-free number developed by ChildHelp.org and the O.U.R. Children's Project specifically for Deaf and hard-of-hearing children.

2. O.U.R. Children's Safety Project of Hands & Voices. Hands & Voices is an organization for parents of children who are deaf. O.U.R is a community of parents and professionals who are learning to enhance the safety and success of children with disabilities. It is a community for which silence is not an option. A community that recognizes risks that our children face and are working to reduce those risks.

3. *Do? Tell!: Kids Against Child Abuse* a DVD from The Greater Hartford Children's Advocacy Center at St. Francis in Connecticut. Great for explaining to children what abuse is and what to do. It is about deaf children and *for* deaf children AND all in sign language as well as audio.

4. SB594 is the bill that became law in Tennessee. It outlines a procedure that law enforcement can use to access interpreters on the spot, in the field.

5. Sign Club Starter Kit by Sign Club Co. This is a packaged program to help adults, wherever they may be, to jumpstart a Sign Club in their communities so that their communities can begin learning sign language, learning Deaf culture, and becoming involved with the Deaf in the community. It is easy, fun, and effective. It helps schools, businesses, children's reading scores, and abused children. Launch date is set for Summer of 2017. Sign Camp kits to follow.

Sign Club Co.
142 Imperial Blvd.
Hendersonville, TN 37075
615-838-3876
signclubco@gmail.com
www.signclubco.org
Facebook: Sign Club Co.

6. My Tried and True Favorites:

a. *Through Deaf Eyes*, a DVD. A PBS documentary that I show as often as possible to classes I teach. It is fun, informative, and hits numerous aspects of the Deaf experience from various perspectives. It doesn't pick a side – it just reports the facts.

b. *In This Sign.* This book is a history book by Joanne Greenberg that was later made into a Hallmark movie called *Love is Never Silent*. It is a classic story of what life is like from the Deaf perspective and the CODA perspective.

c. *Raising and Educating a Deaf Child* by Marc Marschark. I read the first edition of this and wrote "Amen!" down the margins as I read it. It, too, provides research unbiasedly.

d. *The Book of Choice.* Leeanne Seaver, ed. This is another great resource from Hands & Voices. I have distributed every copy I had within the first week of purchasing them. Parents need to know what options there are and how to go about making decisions for their children.

e. The Bravo series. A.k.a., Beginning ASL Video Course. This curriculum for sign language instruction is listed in the catalog of Sign Enhancers. It is known as the Bravo series because it features the Bravo family. Students go through daily life with the family: at the grocery store, getting ready in the morning, looking for a remote control, etc. I recommend this for more formal classroom sign language instruction. It is real people using the real language in practical conversations.

f. *Ice Age 4* on Blu-ray has interpreters in the bottom corner...like we used to see growing up. I find this helpful for our kids learning sign language as well as our kids who aren't reading so well or old enough to be reading. They can all enjoy the movie.

7. Other good ones:
a. *A Place of Their Own* by John Vickrey Van Cleve and Barry Crouch. It is a history of the deaf written by the deaf. This history book, this one is a pleasure to read. It isn't thick or heavy, but informative and enlightening. It helps answer a lot of questions that the hearing world have about the deaf world.

b. *Gallaudet's Survival Guide to Signing.* This is a pocket-sized dictionary of the 500 most used signs. It is cost effective and you can carry it in your pocket for handy reference even when you don't have cell phone service to access your apps.

DeafHope
470 27th St
Oakland, CA 94612
510-267-8800 (V/TTY)
510-735-8553 (VP)
1-510-740-0946 (Fax)
Email: DeafHope@deaf-hope.org
Get Help Now: hotline@deaf-hope.org
Business/Donation Info: deafhope@deaf-hope.org
Website: www.deaf-hope.org

Peace Over Violence – Deaf, Disabled & Elder Services
213-955-9090 (V)
866-947-8684 (VP)
866-824-9907 (VP)
213-955-9093 (Fax)
Email: peggie@peaceoverviolence.org
Website: www.peaceoverviolence.org

Deaf Survivor Advocacy for Empowerment (under NorCal Services for Deaf/HH)
4708 Roseville Road, Suite 111
North Highlands, CA 95660
916-993-3393 (direct/VP)
800-799-7233 (Voice after hours)
Email: cmichaels@norcalcenter.org
Website: www.norcalcenter.org/deafsafe

Colorado
Deaf Overcoming Violence through Empowerment
PO Box 150449
Denver, CO 80215
24 hour TTY/Voice Crisis Line: (303) 831-7874 (VP/V) | Hotline@ deafdove.org

Office: (303) 831-7932 (VP/V)
Fax: (303) 831-4092
E-mail: info@deafdove.org
Website: www.deafdove.org

Illinois

Chicago Hearing Society – Domestic Violence Program
2001 N Clybourn Ave
Chicago, IL 60614
1-773-248-9174 (TTY)
1-773-248-9121 (V)
866-932-0167 (VP)
1-773-248-9176 (Fax)
E-mail: AskCHS@anixter.org
Website: www.chicagohearingsociety.org

Iowa

Deaf Iowans Against Abuse
1642 42nd St NE Suite D
Cedar Rapids, IA 52402
319-531-7717 (VP)
319-294-4183 (Fax)
Crisis Hotline V/VP: 319-531-7719
Crisis Hotline (Text Only): 515-867-8177
Crisis Hotline Email: DIAAHELP@c-s-d.org
Website: www.csddiaa.org

Minnesota

Communication Service for the Deaf, CSD of Minnesota
2800 Rice Street
Saint Paul, MN 55113
VP: 651-964-2051
Text Hotline: 651-403-9431
Fax: 651-256-1053
Email: jfrank@c-s-d.org
Website: www.c-s-d.org

Massachusetts
Our Deaf Survivors Center, Inc (ODSC)
PO Box 2276
Worcester, MA 01613
Hotline: 844.637.2723 M-S from 5pm to 9am
Website: http://odscunity.blogspot.com/

New York
ASADV- Rochester Advocacy Services for Deaf Victims
PO Box 20023
Rochester, NY 14602-0023
VP: 585-286-2713
Email: asadvhope@gmail.com
Website: www.asadv.org

Barrier Free Living's Non-Residential Domestic Violence Program
P.O Box 20799
New York, New York 10009
VP: 646-350-2662
Fax: 212-673-5167
E-mail: Nicolynp@bflnyc.org
Hotline: (212) 533-4358 (V); After 5 P.M: (866) 689-4357
Website: www.bflnyc.org

Vera House, Inc.
6181 Thompson Road, Suite 100
Syracuse, NY 13206
Phone: 315-425-0818
24-hour Crisis and Support Lines:
315-468-3260 Domestic Violence
315-422-7273 Rape & Sexual Assault
TTY: 315-484-7263 (business hours)

Ohio
Deaf Women Against Violence Everywhere
PO Box 1286
Worthington, OH 43085
VP: 614-678-5476
Email: info@dwaveohio.org
Website: www.dwaveohio.org

Texas

Safe Place
PO Box 19454
Austin, TX 78760
Email: Info@SafePlace.org
Staff: Deafservices@SafePlace.org
24-hour hotline: 512-267-SAFE (7233)
TTY: 512-927-9616
Website: www.SafePlace.org

Utah

SLCAD – Salt Lake City Sego Lily Center for the Abused Deaf
452 East 3900 South
Salt Lake City, UT 84107
VP: 801-590-4920
TTY/V: 801-997-0452
Email: info@slcad.org
Website: www.slcad.org

Vermont

Deaf Victims Advocacy Services
PO Box 61
South Barre, VT 05670
VP/V: 720-235-6539
Fax:1-802-479-9446
Email: kdarling@dvas.org
Website: www.dvas.org

Washington, DC

DAWN – Deaf Abused Women's Network
5321 First Pl NE
Washington, DC 20011
Hotline 24/7 Pager: hotline@deafdawn.org
VP: 202-559-65366
Fax: 1-202-466-3226
Email: info@deafdawn.org
Website: www.deafdawn.org

Wisconsin

Deaf Unity
PO Box 8713
Madison, WI 53708
Hotline email: help@deafunitywi.org
VP: 608-467-8084
Email: deafunity@gmail.com
Website: www.deafunitywi.org

Bibliography

ADWAS, Abused Deaf Women's Advocacy Services. Retrieved February 26, 2016.
www.adwas.org/information/domesticviolence/

Babcock, Maltbie D. (1901). "This Is My Father's World" in *Praise for the Lord*. Ed.
John P. Wiegand. (Nashville: Praise Press, 1997) 669.

Cook, P. (2007). White Ape. *Terps! And Tales from Deaf Culture*. PC Productions, Chicago, IL.

DeArmond, Lizzie (1916). "O the Things We May Do" in *Praise for the Lord*. Ed. John P. Wiegand. (Nashville: Praise Press, 1997) 497.

Do? Tell!: Kids Against Child Abuse (2007). Dir. Leslie Warren. The Greater Hartford Children's Advocacy Center at Saint Francis. DVD.

Gallaudet Research Institute. (December, 2003). Regional and national summary report of data from 2002-2003 annual survey of deaf and hard of hearing children and youth. Washington, DC: GRI, Gallaudet University.

Geers, A. E. (2006). Spoken language in children with cochlear implants. In P.E. Spencer & M. Marschark (Eds.), *Advances in the spoken language development of deaf and hard of hearing children* (pp.244-270). New York: Oxford University Press.

Haack, Larry and Michael Higgins (2015). "The Song You Gave Me." Print.

Heber, Reginald(1819). "From Greenland's Icy Mountains" in Praise for the Lord. Ed. John P. Wiegand. (Nashville: Praise Press, 1997) 161.

Hey, Johann(1837) and Elmer L. Jorgenson(1921). "Can You Count the Stars?" in *Praise for the Lord*. Ed. John P. Wiegand. (Nashville: Praise Press, 1997) 78.

Higgins, Michael (2016). "In This House." Print.

---(2015). "Semicolon." Print.

---(2015). "What It Really Is." Print.

Higgins, Michael and Jeb Stuart Anderson(2015). "Love Ain't Everything." Print.

Higgins, Michael and Benjamin Higgins(2015). "This is the Life." Print.

Higgins, Michael and Benjamin and Emily Higgins (2015). "You Can Ride With Me." Print.

King, Jr., Martin Luther. Letter From a Birmingham Jail. April 16, 1963. Retrieved Feb. 26, 2016. www.africa.upenn.edu/Articles_ Gen/Letter_Birmingham.html

Marschark, Marc (2007). *Raising and Educating a Deaf Child*. New York: Oxford University Press.

Martin, Civilla D. (1906). "His Eye is on the Sparrow" in *Praise for the Lord*. Ed. John P. Wiegand. (Nashville: Praise Press, 1997) 235.

Merrill, William P. (1911). "Rise Up O Men of God" in *Praise for the Lord*. Ed. John P. Wiegand. (Nashville: Praise Press, 1997) 554.

Mitchell, R.E., & Karchmer, M.A. (2004). Chasing the mythical ten percent: Parental hearing status of deaf and hard of hearing students in the United States. *Sign Language Studies*, 4, 138-163.

Nadi, Aliza. "National Deaf Academy, Hit Wit Abuse Allegations, is Closing." *NBC News*. Jan. 15, 2016. Web. Retrieved Feb. 28, 2016. http://www.nbcnews.com/news/us-news/national-deaf-academy-hit-abuse-allegations-closing-n497516

National Child Traumatic Stress Network. (October, 2006). Deaf children have higher rates of sexual abuse and inadequate treatment: White paper seeks to bridge treatment gaps. Los Angeles: National Center for Child Traumatic Stress. www.nctsnet.org

Rey, Maude L. (1903). "My Task" in *Praise for the Lord*. Ed. John P. Wiegand. (Nashville: Praise Press, 1997) 446.

Sherwin, William F.(1869). "Sound the Battle Cry" in *Praise for the Lord*. Ed. John P. Wiegand. (Nashville: Praise Press, 1997) 594.
Simon, Paul and Art Garfunkel (1964). "The Sounds of Silence." *Wednesday Morning, 3AM*. Simon and Garfunkel. CBS. Vinyl Recording.

Stone, Samuel J.(1866). "The Church's One Foundation" in *Praise for the Lord*. Ed.John P. Wiegand. (Nashville: Praise Press, 1997) 624.

Traxler, C.B. (2000). Measuring up to performance standards in reading and mathematics: Achievement of selected deaf and hard-of-hearing students in the national norming of the 9th Edition Stanford Achievement Test. Journal of *Deaf Studies and Deaf Education*, 5, 337-348.

Acknowledgments

This work is a product of so many people's stories. Thank you to the children and adults who have stayed strong and grown despite the abuse. Thank you to the interpreters who have loved and helped these children and endured so much heartache for these children. Thank you to the Deaf Education teachers who have fought the good fight and the administrators who have held strong.

Thank you to Jamie and Ryan for getting these stories off the shelf. Thank you to Tena, Tami, Connie, Rose, Mike, Beth, Sharon, Phillip and Sylvya for having my back.

I must send a huge thank you to my parents who first loved the Deaf and worked decades side by side with them.

Thank you to my sweet prayer warriors who put on the armor with me every day.

And without my dearest, loving husband and two precious girls, this would not be. They have endured a fight that was not theirs to fight. They have suffered and gone without so that others might be safe. I love you and I thank you.

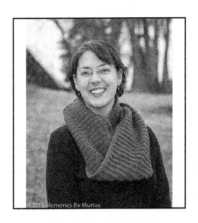

POPPY O'GUIN STEELE

Poppy O'Guin Steele is the founder and Executive Director of the Sign Club Co. which teaches sign language to children and advocates for abused Deaf children. Poppy married her high school sweetheart, and they have two grown daughters. The family enjoys music, traveling, hiking and roasting marshmallows around the campfire.

CPSIA information can be obtained at www.ICGtesting.com
Printed in the USA
BVOW08s0231280316

441983BV00004B/112/P

9 781942 905356